Simple Human Compassion

Simple Human Compassion

The End of Life Craves Touch, Not Technology

by Rick Schneider

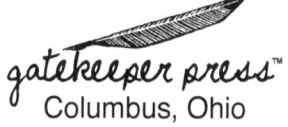

gatekeeper press
Columbus, Ohio

The views and opinions expressed in this book are solely those of the author and do not reflect the views or opinions of Gatekeeper Press. Gatekeeper Press is not to be held responsible for and expressly disclaims responsibility of the content herein.

Simple Human Compassion: The End of Life Craves Touch, Not Technology

Published by Gatekeeper Press
2167 Stringtown Rd, Suite 109
Columbus, OH 43123-2989
www.GatekeeperPress.com

Copyright © 2022 by Rick Schneider

All rights reserved. Neither this book, nor any parts within it may be sold or reproduced in any form or by any electronic or mechanical means, including information storage and retrieval systems, without permission in writing from the author. The only exception is by a reviewer, who may quote short excerpts in a review.

Although this publication is designed to provide accurate information regarding the subject matter covered, the publisher and the author assume no responsibility for errors, inaccuracies, omissions, or any other inconsistencies herein. This publication is meant as a source of valuable information for the reader, however it is not meant as a replacement for direct expert assistance. If such level of assistance is required, the services of a competent professional should be sought.

Library of Congress Control Number: 2021952042

ISBN (paperback): 9781662920493
eISBN: 9781662920509

Author Contact information:
Rick Schneider
PO Box 594
Lancaster, Ohio
43130

Rickschneider-Author.blogspot.com
rickschneiderauthor@gmail.com
740-475-8824

Dedication

WITH LOVE I dedicate this book to my wife, Vickie, whose 32-year nursing career was spent caring for residents in nursing homes. Her quiet presence and care to those in the last hours of their life has always been an inspiration to me. Her example brought me to hospice.

Contents

Acknowledgements xi
Foreword xvii
Introduction 1

Chapter 1: Thinking About It 5
    Peace Begins 6
    We Don't Make it Worse 7
    Don't Go There 9
    Hospice is Stories 10
    No Place Like Home 12
    Not the Answer I Wanted 16
    The Family is Included 19
    Same Boat, Different Oars 21
    Absence of Judgment 22
    The Purest Love 23
    We're Not Just for Cancer 26
    Two Myths 28
    A Much Better Life 30
    A Great Big Hug 31
    They Are Wonderful 32
    A Much Better Experience 34
    After the First Call 36

    Do I Have to Die? 40
    How is Everything in Eastchester? 41
    The Call 45
    A Person or a Patient 46
    Choices, Not Restrictions 48
    How We Face the Last Stage of Life 50
    The Best Things in Life 54
    A Very Common Myth 56
    No Two Alike 58
    So Thankful They Asked 60
    On Her Terms 61
    The I in Team 62
    At the Fair 64
    A Wrench for Every Nut 66
    From the Family's Perspective 68
    I am a Normal Person 72
    Some Things I Cannot Change 74
    Your Family Doctor 77
    The Life Business 80
    The Bitter End 82

Chapter 2: Experiencing Hospice 85
    There Are No Dumb Questions 86
    Thy Will Be Done 90
    Fur Instead of Wings 92
    A Wonderful Fall Wedding 96
    An Order of Fried Chicken 99
    Basic Nursing 103
    Holding Hands 105
    Not a Medical Event 107
    Where's the Other Sock? 108

Mom's Favorite Color 109
Nothing is Insignificant 110
The Importance of Place 111
Our Bedside Staff 112
Beyond the Person in the Bed 116
All You Have to Do Is Ask 120
Custard from Heaven 121
Peanut Butter and Banana Sandwich, Coming Up 124
Chester, Our Cat 126
Pets are Included 128
Pets Can Be A Part of the Plan 132
Even Cats Sometimes Help 135
Dogs Just Know 137
True Comfort 139
A Metal Folding Chair 140
Not Around When Not Needed 143
Do Something with That Hair 144
Graduations 148
She Left as She Came 152
Celebrating the Lasts 154
A Freeing Experience 157
It is Spiritual 159

Chapter 3: The Ache Begins 163
This Gift is from My Sister 164
Where She Needed to Be 168
A Thank-You Card 170
Daylight Saving Time in Heaven 171
How Do You Do This? 172
And Then Some 174
Come Be With Me 176

Chapter 4: A Culture of Kindness **179**
    A Dad of Few Words 180
    His Donation 182
    February is Heart Month 184
    Celebrate Independence 187
    The County Fair 190
    Christmas Angels 193
    Attention on the Midway 194
    Giving Your Heart to Another 195
    Military Pinning Service 197
    Veterans and Their Families 199
    The Simple Act of Showing Up 203
    Burnt Cheeks 205
    A Grilled Cheese Sandwich 206
    And Palliative Care 208
    Enjoyable and Satisfying 210
    The Camel 213
    What Does a Nursing Assistant Do? 215
    Alone No More 220

Chapter 5: When Death Approaches **223**
    The Conclusion of Life 224

Glossary 228
Request for personal experiences 235
Index 237

Acknowledgements

FROM THE FIRST day of deciding which of my written articles to include in this book to the point of telling the printer to "let 'er rip," it has been a labor of love. "Labor" lets you know it took quite an effort; an effort that included many. I want to acknowledge the following who contributed to the completion of *Simple Human Compassion*. Without their help this book would never have been actualized.

I've learned the hard way that an author never edits his or her own writing. In my writing I have relied upon and owe a large debt of gratitude to Susan Foglesong. She has edited and critiqued my newspaper columns for many years. As a hospice employee she understands the philosophy of hospice care and her editing reflects that insight. Even with a busy schedule, she was deeply involved in the editing of this book. I must also acknowledge Susan's patience for the many times she came to my rescue by finding a document I lost somewhere in the computer or explaining, again, how Dropbox works.

I must recognize Denise Bauer RN RRT CHPN, retired CEO of FAIRHOPE and Palliative Care, Inc. in Lancaster, Ohio. The "feeling" of a hospice organization starts at the top and filters down. In her tenure, she raised an already high standard of service and reaffirmed the culture of kindness the philosophy of hospice encourages. The vast majority of the stories in *Simple Human Compassion* would not have occurred if not for her understanding of that philosophy and allowing it to blossom.

And I need to thank Kristin Glasure LSW APHSW-C who took a chance in January, 1997 and accepted my application to be a hospice volunteer. That seemingly insignificant act set the stage for the most rewarding career I could have ever imagined. At that time, she was our social worker and our volunteer supervisor. She is now FAIRHOPE Hospice's CEO. Her devotion to the hospice philosophy of care and to those on hospice service is demonstrated by the fact that she told me about the incident behind the story "True Comfort" found in this book.

Special thanks to Twylia Summers FAIRHOPE's Volunteer Manager. Beginning as a volunteer during the same period I did, she is now our Volunteer Manager. Twylia has made suggestions and made me aware of interesting situations our volunteers have experienced. Quite a few stories contained in this book have her touch on them.

A special thank you to Alyssa Barnecut, owner of Alyssa Barnecut Designs, for her work in designing the book cover. Her creativity coupled with her understanding of the hospice philosophy of care resulted in a book cover that, even before the book is opened, conveys a reassuring feeling that it will bring comfort.

Donna Menigat, a noted local amateur photographer, and fellow hospice volunteer was also involved with the book cover. Donna used her God-given talents to take the beautiful photo used in the cover art and the author photo on the back cover. Additionally, she was a member of the group who helped narrow down the large amount of title suggestions to a short list of finalists. Thank you, Donna.

Thank you to Nancy Henry MSW LSW APHSW-C for her

suggested subtle enhancements to the book cover appearance, conversations with me regarding our military pinning service and her on going encouragement throughout the completion of this book.

Fred Menigat, who was also in the book title group and is the handsome male model on the front cover. I wonder if during the photo session he heard, "Just one more". And speaking of the book cover, I need to give a special thank you to Ellen, who stole the show on the front cover.

I need to recognize one of my favorite people at FAIRHOPE who, by coincidence, happens to be a highly respected baker, Linda Foglesong. "Custard From Heaven" is an example of Linda's intuition as to when a casual remark about a favorite food is in reality a one-last-time desire.

I am deeply indebted to my Gatekeeper Press team. In particular, to my Author Manager Jennifer Clark who patiently addressed all of my concerns, some of them twice, when I forgot that I asked her the first time. Yet, she kept everything moving from start to finish. I'd like to express my gratitude to Rob Price, President of Gatekeeper Press who, whether he knows it or not, changed my idea of publishing a book from, "One day" to "Day One." Also, I owe a debt of gratitude to the whole Gatekeeper Press team for their bringing this book to completion with such outstanding quality.

Thank you to Anthony Penrose RN, for his review of medical terms, words and phrases; ensuring their accuracy.

The COVID-19 restrictions of 2020/2021 forced our hospice volunteer program to be temporarily suspended. One of the adjustments that resulted was the need to have paid staff work at the reception desk of our hospice house. As a paid employee during that twelve month period I worked a weekly part time schedule at the facility's reception desk allowing me to witness firsthand what our nurses, aides and overnight on-call nurses achieve to make our hospice/

inpatient facility, the Pickering House, such a wonderful place. Staff members include hospice nurses: Heidi P., Amber M., Mitch C., Philena B., Shawnna B., Julie S., Heather H., Jayde L., Lisa D., Alma A., Tamera H., and Shelli B.

During my hours spent at the front desk Julie Salyers RN CHPN opened my eyes to the intensity of emotions experienced by the facility's medical staff. In that same vein, Heidi Perkins RN CHPN has been an excellent resource for me to understand the different environments experienced by a hospice inpatient facility nurse versus a home visit nurse. Their touch is peppered throughout the stories in this book.

So many of the stories contained in this book are the result of the alertness of FAIRHOPE Hospice's STNAs (State Tested Nursing Assistants). They are the foundation of the hospice philosophy. Those STNAs include: Stephanie Singleton, Carla M., Traci H., Patsy M., Andrea VB., Madison B., Jennifer J., Sarah G., Lisa T., Madison R., Heather S., Ashley R., Shelly W. Their commitment, love and empathy to those in the greatest crisis in life are valued and valuable.

Family members of those who have been on our service have told me of the positive effect our staff has had on them; many of the conversations taking place years after their experience. I regret that I could not mention each of our staff by name.

My appreciation to FAIRHOPE's Grief Support Manager, Tracey Miller, who wrote the story, "Come Be With Me". Tracey has taught me much about the necessity of both verbal and nonverbal communication during the last stage of life. I also wish to thank Ernie Doling, FAIRHOPE's Grief Navigator who wrote, "How do You do This?". His upbeat "Life is good" outlook has been an inspiration to me. I have been blessed to assist Ernie with memorial services, presentations, children's grief camps and support groups.

Special thanks to Kim McPeek LSW. She has told me about several of her experiences including "The Purest Love". And

I wish to thank Kim Shook and Beth Bobinski RN, both of whom exemplified the spirit of hospice described in the story, "This Gift is From My Sister", when they sensed that someone needed to talk and they took the time to listen. And a note of gratitude to Spiritual Care Coordinators Naomi Calkins-Golter, Mark Linn and Kermit Welty, each of whom told me of their experiences and gave insights into the spiritual aspect of hospice care.

I also need to give a special word of gratitude to all of my fellow volunteers at FAIRHOPE Hospice. So many of the stories contained in this book either featured our volunteers or they were quietly present, in the background. A special thanks to volunteer Pat Meldrum who, through written correspondence and many conversations, conveyed to me the inconvenient compassion required of our No One Dies Alone volunteers.

Thank you to Crissy Devine of Web Chick for her wizardry in promoting this book on the Internet and her timely response to my questions. I am eternally grateful to Ed and Esther Heston, for giving me my first opportunity to have my short hospice-oriented vignette, "Something More", regularly published in their county wide newspaper. The accumulation of those newspaper articles resulted in the one-page stories contained in this book. And by the way, Ed, thanks again for your emails reminding me to get the copy to you by deadline.

To Deb Tobin who, as editor of a local newspaper, gave me encouragement and suggestions for my regular column. And to Amy O'Nail and Autumn Warthman, publishers of an area wide publication for making space for my regular column.

To those on my "Title Review Board" who helped to whittle a long list of potential titles down to a few: Lindsey Schneider, Patti Abel, Tim and Lu Fox, Tammy Drobina, and Sr. Janet Schneider CDP. Lindsey also reviewed the first batch of stories to evaluate their subthemes used in the Index.

A special thank you to Ann Hammond for her support and

enthusiasm in promoting my first book and her continued support, and words of encouragement, for this one. To André Clemons, an employee of one of my hospice's non-medical suppliers. His cheerfulness and many insights into life's tribulations were positive motivators for me. And, I might add, his sometimes strained relationship with our cat, Chester, was always a pleasant diversion.

To Rick Bagby, a friend and retired high school English teacher who helped point the *Simple Human Compassion*'s Introduction in the right direction. To Bob Competti for his permission to quote lyrics from his song, "Celebrate My Soul".

A good hospice offers services that others don't. Since Medicare only covers the basics, donations are needed for a hospice to do the little things that impress so much, many detailed in this book. One annual fundraiser that stands out is the Annual Egg Roll Run produced by Ernie Cook. The motorcycle poker run, named after his deceased brother Eddie "Egg Roll" Cook, has become an annual must-go event. Thank you to Ernie and those who have been vital to its success: Dee Stebelton and Teresa Cook, Roseonna Frishette of the Old Town Tavern, and the band, Hillbilly Deluxe. Through their interaction with attendees band members Seth, Devin, Jason, and Zack, have been "instrumental" in the poker run consistently exceeding the previous year's donation.

I apologize for the oversight if I left anyone's name out. All who helped, in any way, were important to the success of *Simple Human Compassion*. Thank you all.

Foreword

MY NAME IS Dr. Maureen Keeley (PhD) and I have been teaching and writing about communication (e.g., interpersonal, family, nonverbal, relational, and end-of-life) for over three decades. More specifically, I have focused my research for the past twenty-two years on communication at the end-of-life, specifically focusing on "Final Conversations" that occur between family members and their loved one that is terminally ill. I have over fifty academic publications, and most importantly, I am co-author with Dr. Julie Yingling for the award-winning book *Final Conversations: Helping the Living and the Dying Talk to Each Other* (2007). I have just been honored with the national "Bernard J. Brommel Award" (2021) for Distinguished Family Communication Scholarship for my body of work on communication at the end-of-life. I am giving you this brief background of who I am, and highlighting my expertise, because I believe that I can bear witness to the outstanding quality and importance of Rick Schneider's book *Simple Human Compassion: The End of Life Craves Touch Not Technology*. This is a brilliant, heart-warming, and insightful book full of stories from his experiences as a Hospice Volunteer and as a Hospice Patient-Contact Volunteer, as well as from memories that were shared with him by family members that had a loved one that was cared for in Hospice. This book highlights the care and compassion that Hospice offers to the dying and their family members.

Understandably, for many people there are a lot of negative emotions (e.g., sadness, fear, and anger) around death and dying; yet somehow the stories shared in this book demonstrate the good that comes out of the experience of walking alongside our loved one on their final journey in life. As the author notes in the chapter *"The Life Business"* Hospice is in the LIFE business because it is their mission to help the family members and their terminally ill loved ones to focus on minimizing pain for their loved one, to take the mystery out of the stages of dying, to share compassion with the family as well as with the dying. It is important to focus on living through the final stages of life rather than trying to avoid it, because by recognizing and embracing everyday actions and routines, people are reminded of what is important—the small things that make up life, such as a good night kiss, holding hands, sharing and laughing at a funny story, eating a meal together, reading bedtime stories, watching a sunrise or a sunset, and so many other simple, daily activities. During this end-of-life journey, family members and their dying loved ones have the opportunity to create new memories and reminisce about past memories, prioritize their relationship and share precious time with one another, celebrate each other's accomplishments as well as their relationship, and ultimately connect through words, touch, and a final look.

"Simple Human Compassion: The End of Life Craves Touch Not Technology" is not a preachy self-help book, it is a storybook filled with love and compassion, it is a book that highlights the importance of communication, touch, and showing up for their loved ones' final journey. Everyone needs help when they come into this world and they need help to leave it, everyone wants a witness to their lives, to be reminded that they made a

difference during their lifetime, and it is this human connection at the end-of-life created through words and touch that will keep the family members company long after their loved one has died.

I highly recommend *Simple Human Compassion: The End of Life Craves Touch Not Technology* because it focuses on the people and not the disease. It allows the reader to recognize themselves, to address their unspoken fears about death and dying in an unthreatening way; it embraces the physical, emotional, mental, and spiritual journey at the end-of-life. Rick Schneider and I share a common goal, we want people to communicate at the end-of-life for the benefit of everyone involved. I applaud Mr. Schneider's work and I invite you to join us on this journey.

—Maureen P. Keeley, Ph.D.
Professor of Communication
Texas State University

If you want a happy ending that depends, of course,
on where you stop your story.
—*Orson Welles*

Introduction

"What else can I do?" is a question often asked in frustration when a loved one's treatments aren't having any effect on slowing a disease's progress, and there seems to be nowhere to turn. For some, the seriousness of an illness is denied and only dawns on them slowly over time. The ensuing emotional strain is a load you can only carry if you have help. The good news is help is available and can be as effortless as *Simple Human Compassion*.

The book you are holding offers many examples of a comforting, gentle option that is available when there appear to be no other options. *Simple Human Compassion* may just end up as a comforting, gentle option for you as well. It presents easy-to-understand information when the time arrives to make very difficult decisions. Much of hospice care involves just plain old common sense.

The book may be read in any order, logically progressing from defining the hospice philosophy of care to touching on grief. Reading this book will give insight to help you when making the decision as to whether to call hospice or not.

Sometimes in the last stage of life, what needs to be healed is the mind, not the body. As you choose different stories to read, your eyes will be opened to the normalcy and humanness of the hospice philosophy of care, of how it is able to bring calmness, and even serenity, to a dreaded situation. Throughout, you will realize it is the terminal illness, not hospice care, that is the culprit.

I understand that almost everyone who is buying this book is, for any one of many reasons, concerned about the end of life. And from my experience, the interest isn't as much in gaining overall knowledge about the end of life as it is finding relief from current emotional distress. Therefore, I've kept the stories in *Simple Human Compassion* relatively short and to the point, many only one page in length. The book is easy to read, and information is easy to find.

During my twenty-four-plus years of being a hospice patient-contact volunteer, I've learned that we care for people, not patients. Yes, by necessity, anyone under any sort of professional physical/mental care is referred to by the generic word "patient." The hospice philosophy subliminally returns the patient back to being a person. In *Simple Human Compassion*, I refer to those on hospice service as people who are ill. Not as patients.

As you read this book, you will learn that the hospice philosophy of care is not a template of procedures but more of a comforting service. Medicine in the hospice setting is generally used for physical comfort, but hospice also addresses the need for emotional and spiritual comfort. A good example of how emotional comfort in the hospice setting is received is demonstrated in the story "A Wonderful Fall Wedding." It beautifully describes how the mother in the story still had purpose in her life, which gave her emotional comfort, even at the very end of her life.

Ever since I became a hospice patient-contact volunteer, the comments from someone who has witnessed hospice's compassionate care invariably include, "If only I knew." By relating to my experiences through a wide variety of stories, you will understand why that comment is so common. It may seem to be contradictory, but hospice is a philosophy of care focused on living life to its fullest. The hospice philosophy of care shows that dying is not synonymous with useless.

Simple Human Compassion will become a reference for you should you or someone you love be confronted with the biggest crisis imaginable. The index directs you to the pages containing answers to your specific questions. Inside, you will find answers to myriad questions, ranging from acceptance of the situation to the Medicare requirement for volunteers in hospice.

The answers may be presented either directly or indirectly. For example, the story "Where's the Other Sock?" is about an experience I had as a volunteer doing the laundry of a person on service. The story takes place in the person's home and conveys two ideas: first, hospice philosophy provides care for people where they live. And second, volunteers help bring normalcy back to life, and doing laundry is as basic as it gets. Not to ruin the end of the story, but, yes, we came up one sock short.

In March 1997, when I began my career as a patient-contact volunteer with FAIRHOPE Hospice and Palliative Care, Inc. in Lancaster, Ohio, I was then, and still am today, enthralled by what we do in the hospice field. As of July 2021, I have accepted a little over one hundred and seventy patient-contact assignments. I also volunteer as a member of our No One Dies Alone program and am a member of our Military Pinning program. My comprehensive experience includes being present at several consults as the family was having intense discussions about their parent's immediate future.

On the other end, I have made several "death calls" after the passing of a person on service in his or her home, assisting the family until our nurse could arrive. I have given eulogies and facilitated grief support groups, along with assisting and facilitating memorial services. I have been very fortunate to have experienced everything a hospice organization has to offer.

Frequently, the one who is ill has accepted his or her situation and is preparing for what lies ahead. Conversations from the heart during this time are paramount, and as hospice allows those involved to focus on what is really important, these vital conversations naturally occur.

I want to emphasize, as discussed in the book, that hospice is not a single, universal organization; each hospice is unique in how it meets Medicare guidelines. Therefore, some hospices may not arrange or allow some of the events I describe in this book. The choice is theirs.

I urge you to pick up a copy of *Simple Human Compassion*. Truly, the end of life craves touch, not technology.

CHAPTER 1
Thinking About It

"Some of us think holding on makes us strong, but sometimes it is letting go."

—Hermann Hesse

Peace Begins

I was talking to a friend of mine, and he said the general public's perception of hospice care is that it's a signal of giving up. I guess it is a matter of perspective. Having been associated with hospice, I've witnessed and learned we don't give up on a person's life. We help people embrace it.

One of the subliminal aspects of hospice is how we acknowledge that someone is still alive. We call people by name and don't ask them when they were born every time we see them. We sit with people if they desire, and acknowledge they are still living and that, even now, they have wants. Those wants may be of a physical, emotional, or spiritual nature. We address each one. I might add that the comfort we bring is for both the person on hospice and the individual's family. An incurable disease affects the entire family.

The general consensus, I think, is it appears to be giving up when hospice is called. The family is perceived as giving up on their loved one. Part of this may be due to the lack of information regarding hospice care and also because there is a lifelong familiarity with curative medicine protocol.

During an immense crisis, there is a need for a "business as usual" reassurance, not something new that signifies a familiar process is no longer beneficial. What is important to be understood is that this stage is different from any other stage, and it deserves, actually requires, a new and different manner of care and a new way of approaching life. The last stage of life demands our full attention, with no distractions from technology.

Eventually, expectations of a return to health must be let go. It is not giving up, but a simple, anguishing fact of life.

Peace begins when expectation ends.

We Don't Make it Worse

WHEN PEOPLE TELL me about their experience with hospice, they frequently mention if only they knew what we did, they would have called us sooner. On a few occasions, I've asked people if anything in particular stands out as to what they wish they had known before calling us. Most have a hard time trying to single out anything. Generally, I hear comments saying everything became calmer and more peaceful once hospice was invited to help.

One person, who I think was speaking for many, said, "One of the things that I wish I knew was that hospice didn't continue to make things worse but actually made things better for my family and my dad (the person on service)."

I had not thought about it that way, but he was correct. With Medicare, the ill person pays nothing for basic hospice care. We are required to contact their insurance company, if covered, for payment. We don't make your medical debt worse. All hospices offer a variety of services at no charge and many extra services at a nominal cost. Most hospices don't require you to move into a special facility of any sort, thus reducing your anxiety from all of the disease-driven life changes that have been experienced up to this point.

Hospice doesn't perform any curative treatments. For that reason, we don't distress you with decisions on going through any more surgeries or suffering adverse side effects. We merely allow you and your family to enjoy each other during the remaining time.

We don't make things worse because we don't do what everybody else has already done. I think what it boils down to is, if you can't change your situation, you can at least improve how you deal with it. In hospice, you are the decision maker and can now direct how you wish your care to continue, putting you back in control. During the crisis of your life, please call hospice. We don't make it worse.

Don't Go There

"I'D NEVER SIGN onto hospice; they kill people!" I've heard people say this quite often when discussing hospice care. That same sentence arises when discussing a loved one who has an incurable disease. The idea that any hospice would kill someone just doesn't make sense when you think it through. You really don't have to think it through too far. From just the financial aspect, how do hospices get paid if they kill people? From the legal aspect, why hasn't anyone called the police?

Just so we can put this myth to rest, hospice does not kill people. Whew, that's good to know, isn't it? In fact, all hospices, whether for-profit or nonprofit (such as mine), get a per diem amount of money from Medicare. This means hospices are paid a set amount of money per day for each day a patient is on service. Knowing that, common sense will tell you that the longer a person is on service, the more money a hospice will receive. The irony is that we want those on service to live.

Not only are people not killed on hospice, but they routinely live longer than expected if they are admitted soon after being told they have an estimated six months or fewer of life remaining. Hospice addresses physical, emotional, and spiritual pain. Many studies by insurance companies and the government have shown when patients are pain free and living in their homes, they live longer. As we say in my family, "And that's a fact, Jack."

I know the word "hospice" can generate fear. Rather than have contempt without investigation, talk to someone who has experienced hospice care. During the crisis of a lifetime, we are here to calm you, to reassure families, and to help your loved one live as long as possible in serenity and comfort.

Hospice is Stories

When I'm in a conversation with someone about their hospice experience, they invariably tell me something our staff did for them or their loved one. This is true where I work, but each hospice is unique. Sometimes a hospice may restrict certain activities or not respond to requests. The stories I hear can be long, with frequent smiles throughout the discussion. There have been times when I thought the story I was hearing was about an event that happened recently, while in reality, it happened over twenty years ago. The emotion in people's voices conveys a more recent occurrence than this to me.

One of the reasons hospice is best described through stories is that there isn't a template of care. Each family is unique, as is each situation. Each hospice organization has the freedom to handle a situation or family request in the way it determines is best. Yet, everyone I have spoken to is clearly at peace, considering the circumstances.

The outwardly mundane little things we do for people under our care and their families are usually initiated by an often whimsical comment. When someone on our hospice laments they will not reach a goal or taste a favorite food anymore, the staff and volunteers come together to see how we can make it happen. That is at the center of where these stories come from. Our staff is attentive to these longings and understands a simple comment may be disguising a deep-seated wish.

My purpose in writing about hospice is to convey the goodness of hospice care. And the best way to convey the philosophy of hospice care is through stories. When I talk to anyone regarding their experience with hospice, people invariably begin by telling me of a memorable incident they experienced. It is rarely, if ever, a litany of facts, figures, or third-person narratives. Through my twenty-plus years of experience, I have heard so many heartwarming stories from those who have experienced hospice care with their family or by witnessing a friend's experience. I felt compelled to convince the general public that there can be peace and serenity in the last stage of life. The last stage of life may be spent living life and not simply trying not to die.

Hospice is about family stories. Hospice is about life stories. Hospice *is* stories.

No Place Like Home

Probably what surprises people the most about hospice is our depth of concern for people who are terminal and their families. Hospice care surrounds ill people and their families with support and empathy during a time of intense stress. Over time, as more people experience hospice, more are aware there is help, true help, when the unthinkable is on the horizon.

One of hospice's calling cards is we allow people on service to remain where they currently live, or if feasible, where they would like to live. If people are living in a nursing home, they remain there, and our STNAs and nurses come to the facility and take care of anything related to their terminal illness. We also administer care if they lived in an assisted living community, an apartment, or their house.

If the ill individuals are still alert and oriented when they accept hospice, we follow their wishes. Not surprisingly, one of the most common wishes is to die at home. I would imagine that's because home is familiar and makes people feel most comfortable. Yet, most of us aren't aware of what supporting a family member at home might involve. Over the past years as a patient-contact volunteer, I have been in quite a few homes. One of the lessons I've learned is that caring for a loved one helps caregivers learn to accept what is happening. They are now a part of it and not passive bystanders.

Many have told me they felt a sense of purpose and accomplishment, as they cared for a family member at home. Sometimes the family will create surroundings that reflect the way the person has lived. I was assigned a patient a while ago who built street rods. His family filled his room with 1950s "Bucket T" photos and mementos, plus car magazines from the sixties, old gas station signs, and anything else they could think of. The man loved it. And to be honest, so did I. Many conversations were initiated by looking at his walls.

If you are considering caring for someone at home, there are some basic elements that should be considered. All of these elements can be discussed with your hospice social worker or nurse. The first consideration is to make sure the ill person and those who plan to be the caregivers understand what will be involved. As always, the social worker and case manager (the ill person's primary nurse) will explain everything in detail. We don't leave anyone stranded without support. Some hospices have made arrangements for on-call medical professionals to assist those on their service overnight, while other hospices, such as the one where I work, are always available at any hour of the day or night. In fact, where I work, your call is so important to us that we actually answer when you call.

We also supply families with everything needed to properly care for their loved ones. For example, if necessary, we will provide essential durable medical equipment (DME), such as wheelchairs, walkers, bath seats, shower rails, and hospital beds to help family caregivers safely provide care. Our team can help you understand what resources you need now and what resources you may need in the future. They can further help connect you to other support networks in your community.

When possible, we try to make sure that there is a bedroom on the main floor. It is their house, so the family can locate the temporary quarters where they please. I have been in homes where either the dining room, living room, or even the kitchen were temporarily converted into bedrooms. Any room will do. It is comforting to know that no matter how small or cramped the living arrangements are, we always make it work.

As mentioned, the home-side team, as we call those caring for you where you live, knows that ongoing communication is essential. This dialogue will help to avoid feelings of being alone during a scary time. Many hospices have twenty-four-seven phone coverage, while others may contract after-hours coverage. In the last stage of life, comparable to the first stage, most activity, it would seem, takes place from 4 p.m. to 8 a.m., rarely from 8 a.m. to 4 p.m.

In addition to the home-side care, hospice organizations such as mine offer an in-patient facility, commonly referred to as a hospice house. Some hospices may lease rooms in a nursing facility or hospital. All of these have the same purpose, and that is to provide symptom management if needed and give the caregiver a much-needed break from constant caregiving. Scheduling regular breaks in advance can help to ensure the caregiver has a period of time to look forward to for rest and to regroup.

Sometimes family members find that much of their energy and inspiration used in caring for someone at home comes from the meaningful two-way connection that exists at such an important time. I have had people tell me that initially they were uncomfortable with the thought of their family member dying where they live, the rationale being the space once occupied by the patient will bring back strong reminders of that person, and families may find it hard to imagine living in these spaces after a death occurs.

But through my years of meeting the general public and talking to people in grief support groups, I have not heard anyone express any regret at having the person die at home. That is my experience. You may have different thoughts on the subject. One person told me the end of life was such an intimate family event that no other place would have conveyed that feeling but home.

Most hospices, mine in particular, are very flexible. If a family is uncomfortable with their loved one dying at home, we will bring their loved one to our in-patient facility to allow the occasion to happen there. We serve those on our service, including the family, and if that is what they want, we will do our best to accommodate their wish.

Whatever decision you make about the location for the death of someone close to you, remember there are always options available to you. You can't always anticipate what will happen or exactly when. But, working together as a team, we can make sure the approach you've taken is right for everyone involved. With the support of hospice, personally helping a loved one during this stage of life may be a rewarding and meaningful experience for the family.

At this stage, families may feel overwhelmed from going to medical facilities to visit their loved one. Often they may find this leaves them with very little time for talking, sharing, or sitting quietly with the person who is dying. When caring for someone at home, caregivers have told me how natural it seems and how it helped them feel that everything was going to be okay.

We believe that life starts and ends with family. And there is no better place for the family than home.

Not the Answer I Wanted

My goal in life is to live forever. So far, so good! Although, my kids have told me that I most likely won't live forever. And whether I like it or not, I think they may be proven correct at some point. However, they added that if I haven't grown up by the time I'm fifty, I don't have to grow up. That gave me solace.

Truthfully, there have been a few periods when sometimes it did not feel like I'd live forever as I've been through several extended periods in my life where I have been very sick. During those times, I prayed for healing. I prayed to be brought back to good, if not perfect, health. In the case of my most severe illness, which manifested itself when I was in my fifties, I did get an answer to my prayers. Looking back, I realized the chronic disease was the answer to my prayers, and it was not the one that I had wanted. Maybe you've had a similar experience.

One of the hard facts of life is that prayers aren't always answered in the way we prefer. I read somewhere that if God answered all prayers as we expected, there would be no cemeteries. In my case, before my illness, I used to believe prayer exclusively changed things. But my experience showed me prayer changes me, and I change things. Over time, I've learned to accept God's will.

The serious illness I developed in 2006 was a chronic (meaning lifelong) illness known as Crohn's Disease. When the specialist was trying to determine what was causing my physical distress, he thought it was probably Irritable Bowel Syndrome (IBS). He casually mentioned that it might be Crohn's disease but suspected it was actually IBS. He ordered a few more tests to confirm his hunch.

The specialist explained in layman's terms that IBS can be

taken care of with medication or, if necessary, surgery. Crohn's, however, is a lifelong disease that may be controlled but never cured. During the week, while waiting for tests results to come back, I prayed that I had IBS. That is something that I never thought that I would be praying for, but, considering the alternative, it made sense to me. My prayers for IBS were answered, but the answer was, "No." I had Crohn's, not IBS.

By the time of my diagnosis, I had been associated with hospice for almost ten years. During that span, I had spoken with quite a few people who received that same answer to their prayer for healing, i.e., "No."

I feel what I have learned from God's answer of "no" to my prayer and my Crohn's is that it has helped me relate in some degree to many of those on our service. Granted, it is not a terminal diagnosis, but it completely changed my outlook on life. My daily routine, my diet, and even my plans for the future were all affected. I might add that the diagnosis also had an effect on my family.

A diagnosis of a serious illness can rearrange your whole way of thinking about how much future you have and how it will be spent. When I was in good health before my diagnosis, my future was filled with plans and goals. Once I was given my diagnosis, I felt like I had no control of my life and that the disease controlled me. I half-jokingly considered asking for a refund from my church since I had tithed weekly for years, yet my perceived reward was a chronic illness.

Initially, I denied that I had anything seriously wrong. I knew someone must be mistaken. I had to come to the conclusion that the "someone" was me. I've heard receiving a serious diagnosis, such as mine, compared to an unwelcome guest moving in. It changed my way of life and my plans for the immediate future. I did eventually come to the conclusion that I had to accept my predicament because a chronic illness may be controlled, but it can't be cured.

When God's answer to me was not the answer I wanted, I remember a pastor telling me that maybe the answer wasn't no. Perhaps it was just different from what I prayed for. Luckily, while the answer was not what I wanted, my life has turned out better than I ever dreamed. It encouraged me to improve my diet, and it helped me to relate to some degree with others who have not received the answer they wanted to their prayers.

I found that my life became better when I accepted my predicament and let go of my expectations. Hang in there, and remember that everything is going to be okay.

The Family is Included

THIS MAY BE a bit of an understatement, but when someone is seriously ill, the whole family is affected, not just the patient. For this reason, many hospices encourage all who want to attend the initial consult to do so. This helps prevent any misunderstanding among family members as to what will be involved, i.e., what we do and don't do. Questions are encouraged of all attendees so their concerns and fears can be honestly addressed.

With my hospice, there is no limit as to who may attend. Any decisions in that regard are left up to the family. There are times when as few as two people will attend the consult. The attendees might consist of only the health care power of attorney and the representative from hospice. The person in question is frequently unable to participate, as is repeatedly the case when the symptoms of the person's disease prevent his or her attendance. On the other end of the spectrum, those in attendance may include the spouse, grown kids, siblings, and even Aunt Matilda, if she's up to it.

Hospice recognizes that family is the anchor of a loved one's needs when people are experiencing the rough seas of life. Under hospice's guidance, family members may pitch in to help administer care. In fact, it is the option of the family if they wish to play a major role in their loved one's care, a supporting role, or none at all. Each family understands its members, knows their level of ease or unease, and can identify how to best meet its loved one's own unique needs. Much of the decision depends upon circumstances and comfort level. There is no expectation on the part of hospice.

A terminal illness can tear a family apart, or it can draw them closer, to focus on a common cause. When the family does join together to nurse a family member, a spirit of purpose envelops the family. A unity is created that helps to reduce tension and fear.

We encourage family to be involved because the family is affected by the situation too. Yes, the family is included.

Same Boat, Different Oars

When I first heard the song "Celebrate My Soul" by Breaking In, I was floored. It affected me on so many levels because the song is about life, period. It is about the fears all of us have. Are we accepted? Do we fit in? Do we truly accept those whom we perceive as different? Do we feel uncomfortable in their presence? People at the end of life often experience those same fears. They are sometimes shunned because they make others uncomfortable.

The song begins with the lyrics, "Gotta little bit of love, gotta little bit of life." Those lyrics could help describe what we do in hospice care because we give those on our service a little bit of love. I hear time and time again from those on our hospice that they received much more love from us than they felt at any stage of fighting the illness. Granted, the curative realm of medicine does not have time to sit around and talk, while hospices can take all the time families need.

And, believe it or not, we give those on our hospice a little bit of life. We give a little bit of life by focusing on and enjoying what appears to be the little bit of life remaining. I say *"what appears to be life remaining"* because when someone signs on soon enough, the love we give a person comforts to the point that individuals routinely live longer than anticipated. Some to the point of no longer being appropriate for hospice care.

I am not trying to detract from whom the song was directed to. Rather, I hope I can expand its intended listenership to a much broader audience to show that we are all in the same boat. Some of us just have different oars.

Absence of Judgment

PEOPLE WHO NEED help the most often don't look like people who need it. The first time I became aware of this fact of life was when, as a hospice patient-contact volunteer, I took an assignment for an AIDS patient. Our staff accepted the reality of his disease and how he had contracted it. Nothing was to be assumed or implied. However, most of his extended family and society in general during that time did not share the same sentiment.

Once signed on to hospice service, he was moved back into his home from a facility. Immediately after our nurse established his plan of care, the man's bedroom was prepared with all of the necessary medical equipment and supplies. His social worker made sure all necessary legal documents were completed, and our chaplain reached out with a call. The man's disease's progress was somewhat predictable at that point. To the casual observer, it appeared that everything was in order; however, it was not.

The reality was that the man's parents had a son who had been blatantly rejected by society. For years, both in the news media and in general conversation, the message the parents heard was that their son, and "people like him," were getting what they deserved. The man's mom told me of condescending comments that she would overhear about "those AIDS people" even while she was in the checkout line of a store. It was relentless, and she felt crushed. The dad, with reddening eyes, said that when hospice became involved, a feeling of overpowering, indescribable love descended upon him and his wife.

At its core, the essence of love is the absence of judgment. Whatever your ailment or fear, hospice is here to offer tender care and compassion, always with the absence of judgment.

The Purest Love

There is a saying that when the first child is born, the mother is also born. She never existed before; only the woman existed. Everything begins after the pregnancy is confirmed. So many things are required in order to prepare for the birth. The new mother's schedule fills with doctor visits, getting everything in order, and preparing for the new life. Worries that the child will be okay begin and will follow her through life.

Similarly, toward the end of life, should the mother develop an incurable illness, her life will change dramatically once again. After all of the doctor visits, should she choose hospice soon enough, there is the opportunity to get everything in order. And yes, worries that her children will be okay persist, regardless of their age. Truly, when talking about the beginning of life or the ending of life, there can be many similarities.

Not too long ago, I was talking to one of my hospice's social workers, Kim. In our conversation, she mentioned that no matter the age, when a mother is contemplating accepting hospice's service, there is a very high level of emotion. Kim understands that the acceptance of our service signifies one door closing and another opening in a family's life, just as when they learned of a pregnancy.

Signing onto hospice's compassion begins with what is called a consult. The purpose of the consult is to confirm the person is appropriate for this type of care. An important aspect of the consult is it helps our staff to understand the family.

Kim told me of a recent consult in which she was involved. Preliminary to the visit, she learned that the person she was going to visit, "Anne," was a single mom with two grown daughters. When Kim entered Anne's house, there was no one else there. Kim noticed by the woman's expression that she was in considerable pain. Anne wasn't complaining, but when someone gets to a certain level of pain, there is no concealing it.

Concerned, Kim asked her what was wrong. Anne admitted she was in pain but said that it was of her own doing. It was the result of not taking her pain medicine. Anne explained that she wanted to be off the pain medicine long enough to have a clear mind when discussing the possibility of hospice care. She wanted to shelter her daughters from the traumatic event of signing the hospice forms.

Kim has seen it so many times that even though a mother's children may be middle aged, she still worries about them and tries to protect them. Anne had arranged the consult without telling her children when it would be. In her mind, she had already planned to sign the form accepting our service, and she wanted to be alert enough to understand what was involved. The pain medicine had been making her groggy.

A mother's love never falters, and Anne wanted to save her two daughters the emotional pain of watching her sign the forms. The three of them had already agreed that accepting hospice service was the best thing that could be done. What signing those acceptance papers represented was something that was inevitable. She said it was similar to when it came time to give her oldest daughters' baby clothes away. It was so final. Although, Kim explained, should her disease stabilize or improve, she would have to sign off of hospice. That was something that Anne didn't realize; it was a glimmer of hope.

To reach the point of signing the papers required changing the family's thinking from curative treatment to comfort care. It was a slow, difficult process for Anne's family. But during that process, the terminal diagnosis caused Anne's perspective of life to change, just as the pregnancy "diagnosis" caused her perspective of life to change.

When we are confronted with a medical crisis, we almost

universally attack it with a laid-out plan of action and do at least some internet research on the illness. In short, doing whatever it takes to eliminate the crisis. This seems to be how all of life's major problems are initially dealt with.

In a nutshell, we tend to plan with our head and not our heart. The lucky ones understand that some areas in the last stage of life need to be dealt with through the heart much more than the head; empathy and restraint are essential.

In this case, the mother knew that now she had to focus on making sure that her family would be all right without her. The disease was not her main concern anymore. As her body was changing, her outlook was changing. Her "healthy body" ideas were gone.

After Anne signed on to our service, she phoned her daughters. They were upset that she had allowed herself to endure such pain. But she reminded them that she was in pain when they were born. She didn't mind the pain then, and she didn't mind it now.

Being a part of hospice has allowed me to witness and to hear of the depth of a mother's love for her children. It also has made me think about how much my mom did for me. I think that a mother's love can best be summed up by what Mother Teresa once said: "I have found the paradox that if you love until it hurts, there can be no more hurt, only love."

A mother's love is the purest love.

We're Not Just for Cancer

"Hospice, we're not just for cancer anymore!" That sounds like a catchy new advertising slogan, doesn't it? The fact is hospice care never was just for cancer patients. The hospice philosophy of care is, and always has been, end-of-life care, regardless of the disease or illness.

When the hospice movement developed in the late 1960s, cancer lent itself to hospice care. During that era, a cancer diagnosis was like receiving a one-way ticket because the assumption was that there would be no return trip to health. The different types of cancer each followed their own somewhat predictable path, so it was possible for a physician to give an estimated life expectancy.

Well then, who qualifies for hospice care? The one sentence that admits someone to hospice care is uncomplicated: a person is eligible for hospice when the primary physician feels that if the disease or illness follows its natural course, there are six months or less of life remaining. Notice that no medical condition is mentioned by name. The *only criterion* is the physician's estimate (with a second physician concurring) that there are six months or less of life remaining. And six months is just an educated guess.

The people on service are evaluated at ninety-day and one-hundred-and-eighty-day intervals to confirm that they are still appropriate for hospice care. If, after one hundred and eighty days, they remain appropriate, people may remain on service for an additional thirty days. Evaluation of their condition will then reoccur every thirty days thereafter.

I have read that the national average of people with cancer on hospice service has declined from being the prevalent diagnosis to now under 50 percent. Other than cancer, the balance of those being cared for by hospice suffer from a wide variety of ailments. Dementia is a growing segment of the hospice population, with Alzheimer's disease being most prevalent within that segment.

Whether you or someone you know is struggling with a life-limiting illness of any kind, consider calling hospice. I understand that it is not a pleasant thought, but by calling hospice, you will talk to someone who will listen. We can assist you when any serious illness strikes. We're not just for cancer.

Two Myths

HAVING BEEN ASSOCIATED with hospice for over twenty-four years, I have seen quite a few changes in the realm of end-of-life care. These changes are, for the most part, good. Yet many misconceptions regarding the hospice philosophy of care persist, two of the misconceptions being the belief that hospice is one national organization and the belief that hospice care is expensive.

I want to briefly explain why those two beliefs are myths. First, hospice is not an organization but a philosophy of care. There are thousands of hospices located in the United States. Each is a separate entity; each has its own unique characteristics and quality of care. However, all must meet Medicare guidelines to be eligible to receive Medicare reimbursement.

As far as expensive, I'm not sure what would be considered expensive. Up until the point of calling hospice, there is a good chance that substantial medical bills have been accumulated while fighting a disease. Whether acknowledged or not, that puts a heavy emotional burden on all involved.

There are two types of hospices. One type is nonprofit, while the other type is for profit. All hospices will provide services covered by the Medicare Hospice Benefit at no charge. However, a for-profit hospice and some nonprofits may charge for other services not covered by Medicare.

Hospices that don't charge for any of their services are becoming fewer and fewer. Regarding not charging, one not-often-thought-of advantage is that the hospice has no interest in someone's ability to pay. There is no concern about a pay source. From the initial consult forward, all of the attention of a nonprofit hospice is focused on administering care to the person on service and his or her family. The additional funds required to continue are received through donations and fundraising efforts. Don't be misled; every person under the nonprofit's care receives the same outstanding care and the same superior attention to his or her comfort.

A Much Better Life

Many years ago, I did the unthinkable. I had a problem that I had to confront. Overcoming it seemed impossible. I made a few feeble attempts to rid myself of the problem, but truthfully, I just ignored it. Finally it got to the point that I had no choice but to face it—the problem was taking over my life. That problem was smoking.

I had to face the fact that I was coughing on a regular basis, and I knew that I didn't have a cold but was, indeed, developing something. I was afraid that the "something" might be one of a variety of heart or lung diseases caused by smoking. Once I faced the problem, I knew that the future was going to be unpleasant in one way or another. Either I would have to go through the agony of quitting (which was unthinkable at the time) or go through the agony of fighting a disease later in life. One thing I understood: the agony of quitting was temporary, while the agony of heart or lung disease was permanent.

I've heard not everything that is faced can be changed. However, nothing can be changed until it is faced. As anyone who has quit smoking knows, confronting the problem and enduring the agony of quitting results in a much better life. Much like confronting your problems, hospice can be a hard choice to accept and face. Hospice can give you a much better life when a serious illness presents an unpleasant future. We can help you to enjoy and celebrate life. It begins and ends with you. But nothing can happen until it is faced.

A Great Big Hug

I THOROUGHLY ENJOY BEING at the county fair booth that my hospice sets up every year because I get to talk to so many nice people. Every year I hear stories and get a few hugs from people whom we helped during an extremely stressful period in their life. And, I might add, many of the occurrences they tell me about happened years ago.

One woman in particular told me about the difficulty she had while her dad was in a Columbus, Ohio, area hospital. She said that no one seemed to be in charge. Each doctor or nurse would say that they'd have to confer with someone else to answer a specific question. Her family felt alone.

Eventually the decision was made to call hospice. The woman said everything changed when our nurse met her family at the hospital for the hospice admission. All of a sudden, someone was in charge. To begin, our nurse explained to the family what to expect as the illness progressed. She then said she'd teach them later how to care for their dad. And she answered questions decisively, without saying she would need to find out and call back later.

The woman told me, "After we took the few minutes to sign on, our nurse started making phone calls." The family was amazed.

The hospice nurse arranged for the hospital discharge of the dad, his transportation home, etc. Confusion was quickly brought to order. The family's outlook changed from helplessness to focus. The family was now able to concentrate on the dad and give him the love and care that only a family can give. According to the nurse, it was as if the family "got a great big hug."

If you feel alone and don't know where to turn, call a hospice in your area. It may be able to help, even if it is only to give you a much-needed great big hug of support.

They Are Wonderful

ONE OF OUR nurses, who used to work at a medical facility, told me how heartwarming it was one morning to witness a husband and wife in bed embracing. They were in the Pickering House, and one was comforting the other. They were savoring what was left of their life together as a married couple. The scene was profoundly emotional, spiritual, and good. It was hospice at its best.

When I say I work in the hospice field, I usually get one of two replies similar to: "Your staff is wonderful!" or "How can you do that?" There never seems to be a "that's nice" type of reply. And there is always some emotion tied to the comment. Why is that? Usually, the ones who say we are wonderful have had family or friends experience our kindness and compassion. And the negative replies are from those who haven't experienced us yet.

A good teacher will help students learn by challenging them because humans learn by being presented with and accepting challenges. Our staff is challenged on a daily basis to find the sometimes nonapparent cause of pain in people on our hospice. Physical pain frequently is the expression of emotional or spiritual distress, and that type of pain is often hidden deep inside.

As with all aspects of hospice care, there is a team approach to the care of every person on service. That team approach allows several different areas of care to be combined to serve one person. The areas of care include a nurse aide, LPN (LVN) and RN nurses, and a social worker. A chaplain is included, but his or her involvement may be declined by the person on service or the family. From the initial consult, the family of the person signing on becomes one of the main areas of our concern.

The team approach, with individual areas of expertise all focused on one person, allows for creative solutions to any situation. The three areas of pain at the end of life—physical, emotional, and spiritual—are professionally addressed by someone in that field of expertise. This manner of care allows for pain to be better controlled.

Having been through lengthy bouts of pain myself, I understand that to be pain-free is a wonderful experience. Our staff knows that, and they are wonderful for our patients and their families.

A Much Better Experience

No one ordinarily thinks of calmness when they begin to find themselves in the crisis of a life-threatening illness. Yet from the volume of thank-you cards received at my hospice, and what we hear in conversation, I know that there is a pervasive attitude of gratitude from those who have received our service. Quite a few of the cards reference our aides, STNAs (state-tested nursing assistants), nurses, chaplains, social workers, and volunteers. I don't know if I'd say the family of someone on service had a good time, but it sounds to me like it was a lot better experience than what was expected.

Thinking about those compliments, I wonder if one deep-down reason exists as to why so many people are overwhelmed by hospice's indescribable care. I have written several articles about the innumerable little things the staff of hospice performs. But is there one core reason for the compliments? I don't know.

I do know so much of what we do is subliminal—below the radar, so to speak. If you've fought serious illness during your life, as I have, you may have experienced what seems like a different specialist for every single part of your body. You begin to feel like you are a problem to be fixed, not a person.

One characteristic differentiating hospice from the curative realm of health care is that we see the person on service as a person. One to be comforted, not a problem to be fixed. We see the whole family, not just the individual who is ill. We see people where they live, not in an office.

Maybe there are so many heartfelt compliments because we focus on life, bringing back as much normalcy as possible to those we care for. There is no doubt hospice is generally the best option that can happen when a person is confronted with the worst. As hard as it is to believe, the last stage of life may turn out to be a much better experience than anticipated.

After the First Call

There is a lot of mystery surrounding hospice care. The one aspect I try to impress upon those I meet is that hospice is dedicated to *serving* the dying. We do not lead, nor do we issue orders; we *serve* the dying. Our focus is to bring comfort, and at the end of life, spiritual comfort is paramount.

One of the hallmarks of hospice care is that most of what it does is unique to each individual and his or her family. Therefore, not everything written here applies to everyone who is reading this. We must follow Medicare guidelines in order to receive reimbursement. This means that certain aspects of signing onto hospice must occur, or at least be offered during every hospice admission.

The focus of folks dealing with serious illness up to the point of calling hospice has been fighting an illness. When it is determined there is no cure, the focus for some continues to be, "Will another treatment possibly help?" But, for the ill person, the focus on the illness diminishes, and his or her attention, sometimes subconsciously, changes to the emotional and spiritual realms of life. This is true even if the decision remains to keep fighting the disease. The emotional and spiritual needs will still be there whether addressed or not.

I would like to go back to what starts the ball rolling as far as receiving hospice care. When the news of a terminal illness is first heard, what can the ill person and his or her family expect? And if called, how does hospice assist?

First of all, dying is not a medical event, period. Since dying is a spiritual event, I want to emphasize the spiritual aspect of the admission process. In part of this discussion I will be tiptoeing around the area of spiritual beliefs. Part of what causes some chagrin among those not familiar with end-of-life issues is why we don't make the attempt to convert someone to Christianity while we have a chance. My experience is that you would have to be in the room of someone near death, sensing the spiritually charged atmosphere, to understand. Also, many choose to fight an illness until it is too late to communicate with the person. By that time, any "discussion" is between the person and his or her Creator.

As responsibilities have evolved over the years, so have hospice employee titles sometimes changed. One of the titles for our staff that has changed is the title of "chaplain." Our chaplains are now called "spiritual care coordinators." This is not to be politically correct but rather to be more descriptive of what their duties are. A chaplain historically was concerned with one spiritual belief system, such as Catholicism, Protestantism, or Judaism. In my experience, our spiritual care coordinators have ministered to at least sixteen different belief systems within our southeastern Ohio three-county service area.

Generally, after a person has been admitted to our service, the spiritual care coordinator will call to arrange a visit. It is not uncommon for our spiritual care coordinator to report a visit was declined by the person or family. A visit is not required by Medicare; however, a request to visit must be offered. Sometimes the new person on our service has a church family. If so, we ask if we may contact the pastor. Sometimes we will be asked to call on the family as well, while at other times we won't.

Should people accept spiritual care visits, our spiritual care coordinator will try to find out what brings spiritual comfort to the ill person, asking important questions like what makes the individual peaceful? What makes him or her calm? Then the spiritual care coordinators try to figure out how to facilitate what the ill person said.

Those questions about peace and calmness surprised me. I

thought the purpose of the spiritual care coordinator would be to determine if the ill person was at peace with his or her situation spiritually. In reality, the purpose of the questions is to learn from the ill person. Spiritual care coordinators walk alongside the terminally ill and their families in order to guide them toward peace.

Our spiritual care coordinators may inquire whether the person is experiencing any spiritual pain and what is most important in the person's life. Since the family is always included in the plan of care, a question asked is how the family can help us with the spiritual aspect of the plan of care. Often, they may contact the person's clergy or spiritual leader. Our spiritual care coordinator may also ask the ill person, "What has been your greatest accomplishment?" From that question, the coordinator can find out what really made the person "tick" in his or her life.

The next question often asked is something I would never have thought of: "What is a safe place for you?" Some say it is "... in my mother's arms." For others it is "being alone in the woods." These answers give insight into deciding what can be done to make the person calm.

As you can see, our care plan for each person is individualized. We wish to understand the ill person. We're not trying to be intrusive but rather trying to help people meet their spiritual goals so they can go through this part of their lives serenely. As with every aspect of the hospice philosophy, the spiritual coordinator of each hospice organization develops his or her own initial contact protocol.

When people are told there is nothing more that can be done, they hear that statement as a death sentence. Actually we all have a death sentence. There is a time to be born, and there is a time to die for each of us. What hospice attempts to do during this time is help people and their families accept their particular set of circumstances and find peace.

Many of us have spent our whole lives trying to control our emotions. We may not want others to know what we are honestly thinking. During the last stage of life, everything changes. We begin thinking with our heart, not with our mind. Hospice serves, and truly listens, to those we serve, allowing for peace deep down in their heart. Yes, peace comes from within. It is not an external phenomenon. But nothing can be done until after the first call is made.

Do I Have to Die?

During the initial consult with a family that is considering hospice for their loved one, many questions arise. A very common question asked by the individual contemplating this decision is, "Do I have to die if I'm on hospice?" Simply put, no you don't. Granted, many people do die while on hospice, but it is because they have a terminal illness, not because they signed onto hospice. It is the disease, not hospice, that causes a life to end.

Actually, when we are called soon enough, there is a good chance the ill person may even live longer than expected. It is well documented that when someone agrees to hospice's all-encompassing love and compassion sooner, he or she lives longer than expected. Some of those on hospice have even had their health stabilized to the point of no longer being appropriate for our care and are discharged from service.

One of the reasons I believe people live longer while under hospice care is because we comfort them, not just with medicine, but with thoughtfulness and honest but gentle dialogue. We bring peace and a sense of calm where there may have been discord and tension before. Once an ill person is comfortable, it is much easier to live and not give up on life. People on our hospice have held onto life just to watch the approaching Michigan vs. Ohio State game, finish a crochet project, or complete some other specific purpose in their life.

If you are facing a medical crisis, consider hospice. We don't focus on the end. Our focus is on comfort so you and your family will have time to be together and live.

How is Everything in Eastchester?

As a newly married man, I took a job driving a Yellow Cab in Dayton, Ohio. It was during the first seven months of 1972, and I was still in college. A little after sunset one evening, I was dispatched to the emergency room of Grandview Hospital. The hospital was just northwest of downtown. Picking up a fare at the emergency room of a hospital was standard procedure in the taxi business. Everyone knew where the ER was located at any of the area hospitals. If not, there were plenty of signs directing you to the emergency room.

Pulling up, an attractive woman came out to meet me. She reminded me of Della Street from the *Perry Mason* TV show of the 1950s and 1960s. As she entered the right rear door, she told me, in a very heavy East Coast accent, to take her to the Sheraton Hotel downtown on North Main Street. Since she didn't sound like a local, I asked her where she was from. As I pulled onto Grand Avenue, she told me she had gotten in last night from Eastchester, just upstate from New York City.

"Well, how is everything in Eastchester?" I asked in my cheerful welcome-to-Dayton voice.

"Swell, I guess. Not so good over here. My mother died a little while ago," she shared.

"Oh, I'm sorry to hear that," I replied, completely caught off guard.

Distractedly, she went on to say, "It's not your problem. Don't worry about it. I just wish someone would have let me know sooner."

It was an awkward, silent, few-minute ride of only about six or seven blocks to her hotel. We were almost to the Sheraton when the woman asked, probably to herself, "Why didn't someone at least call me and let me know how ill she was?"

I again gave her my condolences and told her there would be no charge for the ride. I felt compelled to do something, and I saw a free ride as my way to express my sympathy. I didn't know what else to do. Maybe a free ride would help. She insisted on paying, saying it was my tip for being so understanding.

A lot has changed since 1972, and a good bit has stayed the same. People still die in hospitals, and the hospital staff still wants to protect the family from bad news. But now, with the advent of the hospice philosophy of care, there is an option. Luckily, in my opinion, we are now "re-realizing" that life cannot be prolonged forever. As at birth, most families want to be together at death.

After World War II, science and medical technology increasingly overshadowed the old way of thinking. With the new technologies and pharmaceuticals, maybe death wasn't inevitable; maybe it could be prevented. If nothing else, it could be postponed until later. Doctors' orders became supreme. Medical know-how, along with new discoveries in pharmaceuticals, replaced the natural order of life. However, knowledge and technology cannot replace basic human needs. We are slowly conceding there are basic human needs that can't be scientifically or medically removed from life.

How the end of life occurs is more important than most realize. Years before she became seriously ill, my mom was insistent no artificial means be used if she appeared to be near death. She wanted to go when God called for her. When her time came, my siblings and I honored her wish. How she died, I now realize, was also important to us, her children.

I believe one of the reasons hospice receives so many heartfelt compliments is that we supply basic psychological and spiritual needs to the ill person and their family. Needs that technology cannot supply or replace. Throughout history, until the modern era, most people died at home with family nearby. The family had a role in what was happening. They were able to tell family stories, establishing the dying person's legacy to pass on the individual's wisdom from years of experience. There was time to pass on family keepsakes, make amends as needed, find peace with God, and ensure those who were left behind would be okay.

My wife is a nurse, having spent most of her career in nursing homes. Her experience helped my siblings and me after we gathered around Mom's bed as her life was ebbing. My wife encouraged each of us to individually sit at her bedside and let her know we would be okay. I am so grateful I was given the chance. I imagine it gave Mom assurance that we would be okay, and I know it gave me peace. My mom died with all of us at her bedside. Her peaceful end, admittedly very sad, was a blessing to everyone involved.

In the final stage of life, people want to end their life's stories on their own terms. These end-of-life needs that I mentioned above are among life's most important for both the dying and those they leave behind. It is the way modern thinking has tried to deny families this role, out of a desire to protect the family from the unpleasantness of the dying process, that has made hospice so important.

The woman I picked up at Grandview Hospital did not have the chance to say thank you or goodbye to her mom or to assure her that she will be okay. The hospital where the woman's mother died had been built to do everything it could to keep people alive, no matter what. They probably didn't foresee a need to call the children until there was no life left. According to the daughter, that was exactly what they did.

When someone signs onto hospice, one of our compassionate areas of interest is to learn if all family members are aware of the situation with the terminally ill family member. If not, we recommend calls be made to all, even if the end does not appear to be imminent. We understand that the family may have some duties to finish, some fences to mend, and possibly a few funny stories to tell. Even now, I still occasionally think about the woman from Eastchester, NY.

The Call

THERE IT IS! I've got to grab it. No, better not ... got to ... can't. It's probably better to wait until tomorrow; that way I'll have more facts and I'll know more. No sense picking it up now. What's the hurry? I've got to pick it up. But what if I pick it up then find out in a few days that I didn't need to? Nope, can't do it. I'm a fighter, and this is too humiliating. Besides, that thing must weigh a ton. I just can't seem to pick it up.

Picking up the phone and calling hospice is not an easy thing to do. I imagine if the situation presented itself to you, it would be the most difficult thing that you would ever have to do. Following all of the medical office visits, lab work, tests, and waiting rooms, why add one more medical organization with more forms to complete? What good will it do? Overcoming the fear of the first call can seem impossible. There are so many unknowns.

It's been said that fear is the darkroom where negatives are developed. (Younger people may not understand that one.) Fear is not a shortcoming; it is an emotion. It is our reaction to fear that can be the shortcoming.

How do you know when the time has come for you to call hospice? Simply, if it's on your mind, then call us. There is no charge to call. You can't be enrolled on hospice if you are not appropriate. Something else to consider is, if you change your mind after agreeing to hospice compassion, you can revoke or opt out of the service. No questions asked. Invariably, when talking to family members, the biggest regret they have is that they didn't pick up the phone and make the call sooner.

A Person or a Patient

MOST PEOPLE HAVE been referred to as "patients" at some point in their adulthood, just as many of the people who have signed onto hospice have probably been referred to as "patients" for a long time before coming to us. I think that one of the reasons people invariably say, "If only I knew" once they've experienced hospice compassion is the subliminal way we put the "person" back in the patient. We accomplish it by shifting attention away from illness, medicine, and treatments and focusing on life, relationships, and goals.

Our approach is family-oriented, meaning we treat the entire family as the unit of care. During our initial consult, we determine what the ill person wants, not solely what he or she needs. Based upon what people tell us, we develop our plan of care to satisfy those wants as much as possible. It may be as simple as where they want their hospital bed placed if they will be living at home. For example, as a patient-care volunteer, one of the people I visited requested his bed be set up in the living room so he could still be involved in his family's life, with a bonus of being able to wave to his neighbors. Others have wanted to be settled into rooms that are special to them, including the garage.

Those who don't understand hospice care may see someone on our service as still just a patient. It's true that on government and insurance forms, people need to be referred to as patients. Hospice, however, sees the beauty that remains within. We restore a patient back to a person, one whose opinion is listened to and acted upon, a person who still can exert his or her personality.

When the worst crisis of your life arrives, think of seeking the best option you could have, hospice care. Let us care for the person who is ill and his or her family.

Choices, Not Restrictions

My personal experience with a serious illness began around 2004 when I finally decided to go to the doctor to get things "looked at." For at least four months, I had been experiencing a few difficulties I thought would go away, but the pain finally won. My family doctor determined that I had a serious illness and scheduled me to see a few specialists. Soon, either my wife or I seemed to be constantly rearranging our schedules, ordering and picking up prescriptions, or scheduling doctor appointments. My diet became more and more restricted because of my medications and my advancing illness.

Eventually, I realized my life was being controlled by my illness. I had given up a large degree of my freedom. Anyone who has had a serious diagnosis can fill in their own details as to how restricted their life became after their diagnosis and how they began to feel stressed because of it.

Hospice, however, does everything possible to remove all of the restrictions imposed by the disease. In doing so, the stress experienced by ill people and their families is greatly reduced. When people sign onto hospice soon after being given a diagnosis, they are allowed to eat whatever they want and do whatever they are able. If eating is impossible, we will still bring them their favorite foods they may want to have one more time. Ordering something and having it brought to them is one of those things that can be done to make someone feel like a person again.

When people under our care realize a task can no longer be done or a favorite food no longer tastes good, they make the decision to stop, not us. It is now their decision because they are in control. Several years ago, while I was visiting a person on our hospice, he told me while eating a fudge sundae, "Desserts is 'stressed' spelled backward." Hospice offers a life full of desserts, not restrictions.

How We Face
the Last Stage of Life

When told that she would be doing part of her clinicals at a hospice in-patient facility, the nursing student wasn't too thrilled. She said when she first found out where her assignment would be, many thoughts ran through her mind. None of them were good.

"Am I only going to be around old people? Are they all bedridden? Do they have cancer? Can they still talk?" she dreaded. She had to admit her initial thought of hospice was that it would be a depressing place. "After all, don't people go there to die?" She realized all of her thoughts of hospice were negative. She had a case of contempt without investigation, that is, being quick to judge without having all the facts.

As she accompanied the hospice nurse on her rounds, the student became involved in all hospice does, and her impression changed completely. The first thing she learned about most hospice organizations, including the one where she was training, was that people don't go there; hospice comes to them. Meaning hospice is not a building or place. It is a philosophy of care that is brought to where the people need it.

In her own words, the student admitted, "I have come to realize I have never been more wrong about anything." That same response has universally been my experience after talking to someone who has been involved with hospice. "If only I knew" is the comment I hear most commonly from those of the ill person's family members.

As a whole, society's way of thinking about the end of life is changing, just as our nursing student's did. The idea of making the act of dying a medical experience is only decades old. Until the late 1940s, most deaths in the US occurred in the home. By the late 1960s, however, dying had become viewed as a medical event and was no longer treated as a natural or spiritual event. The view of dying came to be seen as something that happened in an institution. By the late 1980s, it was estimated only around 16 percent of Americans were dying in a setting other than a hospital or nursing home.

And that way of thinking of death as a medical event was held by society as a whole. Both doctors and the patients' families seemed to feel that for a seriously ill person, everything possible should be done to prolong life, no matter how much suffering the patient might endure. The thinking was that everyone will die eventually, but we shouldn't let them die now. Actually, that still seems to be many people's way of looking at things when confronted with an end-of-life crisis.

The steady growth of hospice care appears to indicate the general public is starting to understand how hospice care can be a tremendous comfort, especially to the family. Yet, the curative medical field often remains focused on the pursuit of longevity, no matter the cost. There is not much consideration given to quality of life. Quality of life is what the focus of hospice is about. That is where the basic conflict lies.

Hospice allows people on its service to pursue their dreams and have priorities other than simply living longer. We encourage people, with the help of their family, to complete life on their terms and to maintain or fulfill their purpose in life.

In the early 2000s, with the growth of the hospice movement, more books were being written about the modern experience of aging and dying. These books tended to focus on the need for a change of heart regarding medicine's role in achieving higher quality for the dying experience, not just trying to postpone the inevitable.

It is frustrating for hospice staff to see how society's hesitancy to examine the experience of aging and dying has resulted in extended discomfort and suffering. The terminally ill, due to society's seeming denial of death, have been deprived of basic comforts that are needed most at this stage in their lives.

I'm sure there are several factors, but I believe the hospice movement has helped society's thinking to begin to move away from the institutionalized version of aging and death. As with any change, there will be some aversion to a new way of looking at things. Those in the medical field are slowly learning by understanding what works or does not work in the current approach. There is an alternate approach to end-of-life care besides the "do everything" approach.

A physician I spoke to at a health fair told me his impression of what we did was to give a patient a high dose of pain medicine and let nature take its course. His words are what I frequently hear from those in the curative field. "Dope them up" were his exact words. Obviously, that is not true. Hospice's efforts focus on the goal of respecting a person's priorities, allowing people to continue living rather than spending the last six months of life trying not to die. We do everything we can to continue to make life purposeful.

This same physician also mentioned how hard, albeit almost impossible, it is to begin the difficult conversation of telling people, especially someone he's known for a long time, there is no cure for their condition. He said if not the patient, then a close family member will plead that the physician at least try to do something.

The most important aspect during these conversations is for physicians to convey they are on the patients' side, then ask patients about specific fears and what trade-offs they are willing to make. Open discussion allows everyone involved to decide what choices would be best. Hospice is one option.

Not all end-of-life situations are hospice-appropriate. It is very important to look at all sides when faced with the biggest crisis life can offer. But if it gets to the point that enough is enough, consider calling a local hospice.

The student nurse mentioned in the beginning of this column learned through experience how good hospice care can be for many at the end of life. It is the best that can happen when confronted with the worst that can happen.

The Best Things in Life

A FAMOUS FRENCH FASHION designer, Coco Chanel, once said, "The best things in life are free. The second-best things in life are very, very expensive." From a financial standpoint, I think that statement seems to emphasize a big difference between the curative realm of health care and hospice care.

During the most catastrophic crisis of life, the comprehensive approach of hospice care, involving both the people on service and their families, is a tremendous relief. And as with my hospice, along with quite a few others, the care is provided without a focus on a payor source.

Ranking right behind hospice is the often very, very expensive decision to fight the illness to the bitter end. That generally preferred option usually creates a seemingly insurmountable stack of disease-related bills. Looking back over twenty-four years of discussions with quite a few people, I have noticed that those who choose hospice compassion invariably tell stories describing love and serenity when sharing their experience, while those who choose to keep fighting the illness speak of the disease and expense.

In the curative field, there are government agencies available for financial assistance, while basic hospice is reimbursed by Medicare. Also, a growing number of insurance companies now include hospice coverage. The difference between both the basic Medicare reimbursement and insurance income, along with the extra attention given by hospice, creates a financial gap between Medicare reimbursement and expenses. Donations are vital. Nonprofit hospices opt to use donations to cover remaining costs, resulting in free service to the recipient.

A few years ago, a few of the donations to my hospice were

used to purchase an extra-wide bariatric bed normally reserved for obese people. A situation developed where the bed was applied to a nonstandard but very important purpose. Our nurses assisted a man onto the large bed, allowing him to lie next to his terminally ill wife as she was approaching her last hours. The couple was given the chance to complete their sixty-three-year life together as it began, embracing in bed.

This is just one small event that demonstrates that not only are the best things in life free, but with hospice they can be priceless.

A Very Common Myth

There are many myths about hospice care. Most of the myths are a result of not knowing the whole story and, most likely, not wanting to know the whole story. Let's face it, talking about the last stage of life isn't always pleasant. But one of the things I've learned in life is to avoid contempt without examination. I try not to make a judgment about something until I've done a little investigation. So let's do a little investigating into one of the myths about hospice care.

Years ago, probably the first thing that I heard about hospice was, "Don't go there; they kill people." You may have heard or thought the same thing. I still hear of people advising someone not to sign onto hospice because they kill people. There have been stories where "They called in hospice and the next day he died." Truthfully, that does happen sometimes and for one very simple reason: the person was actively dying when hospice was called. For some, the perception of when to call hospice is just that—when someone is in the dying process. Maybe that thought prevails because, if for no other reason, nobody knows what to do when a person is actively dying. It is absolutely a myth that hospice kills people.

And if hospice kills people, then how do they make money? The fact is hospice gets paid a per diem amount of money from Medicare for each patient on service. "Per diem" means "for each day." Sounds like an oxymoron, but we don't want those on our hospice care to die! In fact, many studies by insurance companies, the government, and medical schools consistently show that people live longer on hospice than those spending the last stage of their life enduring more treatments. To ensure a hospice does not try to sign someone on earlier than eligible, Medicare has strict guidelines to ensure someone considering hospice care has a prognosis of six months or less of life remaining. Since we care for people during the last stage of life, yes, many will die on hospice, but they usually live longer than anyone may have guessed.

The truth is that neither my hospice nor any other kills people. We celebrate life. When it is accepted deep down inside, and the only desire is for comfort and serenity, consider hospice care.

No Two Alike

I LIKE TO USE stories and examples to communicate what hospice care involves, but these stories relate to only one hospice, FAIRHOPE Hospice and Palliative Care, Inc. Not all hospices do what we do, because no two hospices are exactly alike. With that in mind, I would like to dispel what, to me, is the number one misconception regarding hospice care, this being that hospice is one national organization. Hospice is not a national organization. Rather, it is a philosophy of care. An organization that provides hospice care is referred to as "a hospice."

All hospices are similar in that each performs the same function of caring for people who are terminally ill, and all hospices are governed by Medicare. However, that is more or less where the similarities end. How care is given is up to each individual hospice. At its core, there are two types of hospices—not-for-profit and for-profit. All hospices offer basic Medicare-required services for no charge, but for-profit hospices generally charge for any non-Medicare-required services. Not-for-profit organizations are less focused on cost and often offer additional services at no charge or at reduced rates.

A not-for-profit has more freedom to do what is necessary to meet the emotional and spiritual needs of a patient, with fewer constraints as to the cost. But these costs must be paid. Fundraising helps hospices with various uncompensated needs. Expenses, including bereavement or grief support follow-up care, are an example of a hospice service not compensated by insurance or Medicare.

All hospices receive a substantial part of their income from Medicare in the form of a per diem rate paid for each person on service. A per diem is a sum of money paid to the hospice for every day a terminally ill person is on their service. The per diem is for basic Medicare-required care expenses, but is generally not sufficient to cover the cost for all expenses. Hospice is not as much a medical-oriented operation as it is a relationship and spiritual organization. Emotional and spiritual needs are intangible and therefore cannot be budgeted into a plan of care.

Besides the funding differences, there is another factor that differentiates hospices from one another. A hospice organization may be what is known as "free-standing" in that it is its own entity, such as FAIRHOPE Hospice and Palliative Care, Inc. in Lancaster, Ohio. Or a hospice may be a part of a larger company that owns a chain of hospices or health-care organizations, in which each location gets direction from their corporate or main office. The larger not-for-profit chains, out of necessity, do tend to be more cost-conscious.

Not to confuse the issue, but there are regional and national organizations that a hospice may belong to, such as the National Hospice and Palliative Care Organization (NHPCO). This may help create the illusion of one big organization, similar to the Red Cross. The NHPCO is a nonprofit membership organization representing hospice and palliative care programs and professionals throughout the United States. It does not govern any hospice. In Ohio, Leading Age Ohio, formerly Midwest Care Alliance, serves the same function for hospices within the state. None of these national or state organizations are governing bodies.

What separates one hospice organization from another is the approach to care for those they serve. To be Medicare-certified, each hospice organization must follow specific regulations, but each organization is free to follow its own manner of how these guidelines are accomplished in providing patient care. Even though no two hospices are exactly the same, one thing is certain: all hospices do much more than anyone expects.

So Thankful They Asked

THE HOSPICE I work for sets up a display in the art hall building of each of the county fairs in our main service area of Fairfield, Hocking, and Perry counties in southeast Ohio. The main purpose for doing this is public awareness. Being visible to the public allows people to become familiar with us and learn what we do. To be honest, not very many people ask what we do for the simple reason that they don't want to know.

Besides public awareness, another purpose for setting up a booth is so anyone who has experienced our compassion is able to personally give thanks for the care given to their loved ones. Listening to the county fair attendees, it becomes obvious that there is a difference in the deep feelings toward curative medicine versus hospice in the last stage of life. I've noticed a somewhat grim tone of voice when the focus of the discussion is fighting the disease, especially if the ill person did not choose hospice. However, when talking to someone about their experience with hospice, people's tone is soft and pleasant.

I've also noticed when someone talks of a loved one who had been fighting an illness to the bitter end, the illness takes center stage. Yet, when people discuss hospice care, the loved one is given center stage. Even without directly telling me, their tone of voice conveys to me that during a time of unthinkable crisis, hospice brought unthinkable calmness.

The people who stop by and talk to us during the fair already know what we do. They are so thankful they asked their doctor for hospice.

On Her Terms

AS AN ILLNESS progresses, there is an invisible threshold that must be crossed when the decision has to be made whether to fight the disease to the bitter end or call hospice. It is important to consider the ill person, and as hard as it is, to let the individual live the remainder of his or her life on his or her terms. While fighting an illness, life is lived on the disease's terms.

Being a hospice employee, I was discussing this subject with a woman who was under our care about how she had come to the point of calling us. She said, for her, enough was enough after over a dozen years of tests, treatments, ambulance runs, and lengthy hospital stays. She said, at first, her family didn't want to discuss it. But she had goals to complete, and the sooner everyone agreed with her desires, the sooner she could get started.

Once under our care, the woman had the pain-free time to give away what she wanted to each family member. The highlight was sitting in her favorite chair, watching the smiles and hearing the giggles as her grandchildren got to open the glass case and pick out their favorite TY© stuffed animals. And one last time, they got to grab a handful of candy out of the always seemingly full candy bowl on their grandmother's table.

She told me after all the hugs, kisses, and "I love you, Grandmas" were over and everyone left, she laid back in her recliner and went to sleep smiling, happy to have given herself the chance to live life on her terms.

The I in Team

"There is no 'I' in team," or so they say. When someone signs onto our hospice, they will soon be realizing, "I am receiving a lot of attention from my hospice's team." With many hospices, someone on service will be assigned a consistent team of the same one or two nurses, a nurse aide, a social worker, and a chaplain. I don't think most realize the importance of having the same people administering the care given during the entire period an individual is on hospice.

The majority of hospices hold regularly scheduled weekly meetings consisting of all the nurse case managers, chaplains, and social workers along with the medical director to talk about new and current people under their care. In my hospice, we meet every Tuesday. We call it our IDT meeting. The letters stand for <u>I</u>nter-<u>D</u>isciplinary <u>T</u>eam. In conversation, it is referred to as our "Team" meeting. We include management staff outside of just those directly delivering care so that every sector of our hospice staff understands the nature of what we do. This may include department heads of each area of our organization and/or office staff and volunteers. The entire organization is in tune with what is being experienced by the direct patient-contact personnel.

Throughout the process of fighting an illness, direct patient care of an individual is scrutinized by a relatively small group of people. Granted, each case is different, but I'm sure most people have not had as many as thirty people listening and possibly offering suggestions on ways to enhance their care. That is what occurs in the Team meeting.

At our Team meeting, we first discuss each person who died the previous week. This provides closure for our team while also providing our grief team with awareness of any family needing additional support along their grief journey. We discuss at length new people who have made the decision to accept hospice care and who have been admitted to our service since last week's meeting. We also talk about those who are temporarily staying at the Pickering House, my hospice's in-patient facility.

If a team member has a concern about one person or family he or she is caring for, the floor is open for discussion. A nice part of our Team meeting is that we also discuss those whose health has stabilized and may no longer qualify for our hospice. It is so nice to "graduate" people from our service. That happens much more often than the general public realizes. In all of these scenarios, our team of chaplains, social workers, nurse aides, and nurses hears about what each member of the team is dealing with and may offer advice or empathy.

During the last stage of life, hospice gives a person more love, respect, and attention than many have experienced in their entire life. One person told me, "I've never been the center of attention before." (He added except when he got in trouble in school.)

With our entire team, the person on service is the nucleus. In my way of thinking, there is an exception to the phrase "There is an 'I' in team" because in hospice you are "the 'I' in team."

At the Fair

I HEAR ON A regular basis that hospice means giving up hope and that the person is going to die. Those who have experienced hospice's compassion know that we focus on living and reclaiming life. We don't focus on the end, but rather on each day. Hospice helps those on service to complete their life, to finish what needs to be finished. We also encourage those we serve to find purpose in their life.

Last year at the Fairfield County Fair, a woman walked up to our display. I asked her if she had any experience with hospice or if she was familiar with hospice in general. She said that she was very familiar because she was currently on our service. What?! I couldn't believe my ears! She explained that she had an incurable illness. She had been given a prognosis of six months, which was why she was on service, but her illness was progressing slower than expected.

She shared that she was regularly attending a support group for her illness. The one thing that she noticed at the group meeting was that she was calm and at peace, while the others in attendance were more worried, anxious, and depressed. She said for her it was a matter of acceptance.

The woman believed that one of the aspects of hospice is that if you sign on when the prognosis is six months or less, and you sign up closer to the six months, we give hope for a purposeful future. Since she had been going to a support group before signing onto hospice, the woman kept attending in order to encourage others in the group. She felt her new mission in life was to share her experience. As ironic as it sounds, signing onto hospice gave her new purpose in life.

Each illness comes with its own set of symptoms and activity restrictions. Some illnesses may give you time to rediscover life and find peace and acceptance. Calling hospice sooner could give you that purpose, and maybe we will see you at the fair.

A Wrench for Every Nut

A FRIEND OF MINE used to say that in life there is a wrench to fit every nut, meaning that there is always someone who knows how to help another, no matter what needs to be fixed. Through the hospice where I volunteer, the variety of people who volunteer, and among the many staff, there always seems to be someone who can help a person on service, no matter what the problem might be.

A while ago a man signed onto our service who could best be described as "hard to get along with." Once he agreed to our service, that was just about the end of any discussion. From that time on, every suggestion or offer to help, whether from our medical, spiritual, or social work staff, was soundly rejected, sometimes even ending with the man slamming the phone down. Often anger and hostility are manifestations of fear.

Our team thought that maybe the man could relate to a patient-contact volunteer, the reason being volunteers have no agenda other than to bring normalcy to what can be a frightening situation. Hospice volunteers are ordinary people who do ordinary things, and sometimes those ordinary things make an immense impact.

Sure enough, one of our male volunteers called the man and said that he just wanted to stop by and say hi. The volunteer happened to have a chronic illness and was able to say the right things during that one phone call. They agreed on a time, and an enjoyable visit was made. As it turned out, the two men were almost the same age, so both had similar "when I was growing up" stories to laugh about. I'm not sure how the volunteer accomplished it, but from there a care plan was developed, and staff visits were made.

Our team had found just the right wrench for this tough

nut. For the remainder of his life, the man, who had been discontented, was now calm and comfortable. This was made possible by finding people he could relate to and feel easy talking with. I have often written about how hospice puts the person back in the patient. And sometimes it can be as simple as an enjoyable conversation with the right person.

From the Family's Perspective

SINCE MARCH 1997, I have been a patient-contact volunteer. When I first began as a volunteer, I was employed full time in the construction business, so I volunteered in the evenings and on weekends. Besides assisting those on our hospice by being a patient-contact volunteer, I loved sitting at our display at all of the county fairs in our service area. When people who had experienced our compassion saw our display, they would usually stop by, share their story, and say thanks.

One of the nice things about being a representative of such a wonderful organization is that I get to hear about the goodness of our care from the family's perspective. Those people who have "Been there, got the T-shirt," so to speak, on what our hospice meant to them when they needed us.

People come up to our display and express their gratitude for the understanding and empathy extended to them, their family, and especially their loved one. In one instance, I was at the Hocking County Fair at our display in the art hall when a woman, whom I'll refer to as "Sarah," came up to thank me. She was grateful for our staff helping her mom, but made a point to tell me that we had also helped the entire family. Her mom had been on our hospice six years ago, but Sarah could still remember everything as if it occurred last week.

Sarah began the conversation by saying she had no previous experience with us. That used to be a common statement. Thankfully, we hear that less frequently as more and more people become familiar with the goodness hospice can bring to a difficult time. Without knowing what to expect, Sarah had been very apprehensive when she made the first call to us.

Sarah was amazed by our attention to not only her mom but the family, as well. She added that her mom's nurse was truly an angel. What this daughter noticed and felt was a calmness and empathy from the nurse. Sarah said the nurse did nothing dramatic or newsworthy. The little, almost unnoticeable things the nurse did were what impressed Sarah. Things like freely giving her time to the family. And "time" is a theme that comes through in so many of the compliments we receive.

In this case, the mom was being cared for in Sarah's home. The nurse took the time to teach Sarah and her siblings special techniques in caring for their mom. Sarah said it was up to them as to how much hands-on care they were comfortable giving their mother. She also remarked on how the nurse made time to spend telling them of other families' situations. She assured them others had been there. "That was very comforting to me," Sarah shared.

Sarah told me that it was so comforting to be assured by the nurse "that our feelings of being scared, overwhelmed, and exhausted were normal."

One of the things that most impressed Sarah was that the nurse took the time to educate the family concerning the normal progression the illness would take through its stages. She revealed, "The information turned out to be such a comfort. That knowledge actually reduced our anxiety. We were now included in Mom's care." Notice that she said "included." To me, that is so much more important than just being "helpers."

Sarah explained how the nurse would sit and talk to her mom. "The nurse got to know Mom so well that she knew how to recognize when Mom was feeling stress. The nurse went to Mom's calling hours after she died. I just never expected that level of love," she told me.

Sarah went on to tell me that FAIRHOPE's entire staff displayed that same level of empathy. She said the home health aide who came to help with her mom's care calmly and patiently taught them how to bathe their mom in such a way that it wouldn't cause her any discomfort. The daughter said, "Because of Mom's disease, sometimes it was hard to move her without causing her pain."

She described our aide as another angel who took as much time as needed to advise them in the best way of caring for their mom and especially the necessity to comfort themselves. On one particular visit, Sarah's mom was not feeling well enough to be bathed, so the aide didn't bathe her. It was just that simple. But she stayed and talked to the family. As Sarah remarked, "She wasn't task-oriented; she was us-oriented."

One night her mom couldn't sleep because of the symptoms of her disease. Sarah related how she called the night-duty nurse. The night nurse could have given her instructions over the phone, but instead, he chose to drive out to their house in the middle of the night to take care of it himself. (Did you realize we also have male nurses?) He wanted to make sure that the medicine would make the family's mom comfortable. Sarah told me, "He sat at her bedside. Occasionally he'd reassure us that Mom was doing much better."

In another example, and at a different fair, I was talking to a woman about the great service we give to families and their loved one. She concurred with what I was saying because we had cared for her father several months earlier. Then, I was sort of caught off guard when she told me that the one thing that really impressed her regarding our staff was that we "weren't there when we weren't needed." I stepped back and had to think about that for a minute.

The woman told me her dad had been being cared for in her home. After about four weeks, he had been taken to the Pickering House in order to give the family a little break from caregiving. She said that one evening at the Pickering House, she and her siblings were "getting Daddy ready for bed." As she continued, she told me the room door was closed, and as her siblings were busy getting their father ready, the door slowly opened. The nurse came in a few feet and stopped. She stood there for a few minutes, then gave a thumbs-up to the family and left.

The woman told me she didn't know what the nurse wanted, but she knew that for their family, taking care of their dad was the most important thing. She said simply, "She just left us alone." This woman went on, sharing that in other situations, the Pickering House staff "only became involved if needed. If we were taking care of Daddy the way we wanted to, they just left us alone."

If you ever find yourself in a situation where calling your area hospice might be one of the options, ask around. Find someone whose family has experienced the compassion hospice can provide to your loved one and your family. Don't take our word for what we do; hear it from the family's perspective.

I am a Normal Person

Life can be good, and it's important to know that it can be good in all of its phases, even in the last stage. A hospice organization, when called soon enough, helps those who accept care to continue enjoying the goodness of life. And part of the goodness of life for many people is interaction with others. Quite frequently the problem becomes family and friends avoiding someone who is terminally ill at a time when many individuals need family and friends. The reasons for avoidance are many. All are understandable.

For those who do visit, there is always that awkwardness of how to start a conversation with someone who is obviously ill and does not have a particularly bright future. One general question I hear is what to say or how to start a conversation with someone who is terminally ill. One person told me, "'Hey, how ya doin?' seems kind of awkward."

My experience has been that the person who is ill already knows that he or she is terminal. One of the people I was assigned to once told me that his terminal illness is the main reason hospice staff stops by his house every few days. "Or, maybe it's because of my good looks," he added with a sardonic smile.

My suggestion when visiting someone who is seriously ill is that you treat the person as you would if he or she weren't seriously ill. Those on our service merely want to go on living their lives as day-to-day as possible. In my hospice volunteer training I was taught to just let the person who is ill bring up the subject if he or she wants to.

A hospice STNA told me one of the people she visits regularly thanked her for talking to her "Like I'm just a person and not someone scary." The individual added, "I am still a normal person."

If you are ever in the predicament where someone dear to you is very ill or terminally ill, and you are hesitant to visit, take a chance and go over. Plan on a short five- or ten-minute stay. You might find out you can talk to the individual as if he or she is, well, a normal person.

Some Things
I Cannot Change

I HAVE FOUND ACCEPTANCE is the answer to all of my problems. Granted, there have been times the answer might not be the one I was hoping for, but when I surrender to a situation or set of circumstances that I cannot change, life gets easier. Sounds pretty simple, doesn't it?

Many people, when told their disease is incurable, become angry. Invariably someone, or everyone, in their family wants to fight it, a noble response being to fight the disease to the bitter end. That is almost everyone's choice.

Several years ago, after months of specialists trying to determine my illness, I was told that I have a chronic illness. This meant it can only be controlled, not cured. As the news sank in, I thought back to an experience I had many years ago. At that time, I worked for a robotics company. It was the early 1980s, and the technology pundits were predicting robots were going to take over the manufacturing world. People were saying that maybe the Jetsons were right after all.

I was excited to be working at a company making robots to be used in the manufacturing of automobiles. This company was even featured in a cable TV documentary about robots of the future. Working in a new company in an emerging field was exciting. I knew my future was secure. After a year, I advanced from working in the parts room to being a buyer. The next stop on my way up was purchasing agent.

On a cold Friday morning in February after arriving at my office, I decided to walk back to the shop floor and check on several component shipments that were due. Everyone was crying. I thought one of our employees had died. I quickly found out just about everyone had been fired. It wasn't a layoff. I soon learned the investors who were financing the company were not getting a quick enough return on their investment. The decision had been made to start over, and over 75 percent of the employees had been let go. Only a few had been asked to stay on to get the company back in shape. There was no mention of being rehired. I felt bad for everyone.

As I was talking to them, I was paged over the loudspeaker to report to the personnel office. I figured I was being demoted from buyer back to the parts room. When I walked into the office, I was handed a pink sheet of paper that said I had fifteen minutes to clean out my desk and leave the building. I was stunned, then angry.

That afternoon, at home on what should have been a busy Friday at work, I was numb. I simply couldn't believe what had happened. Pleading for my job was of no use. The decision had been made by the investors, not my boss. I had to accept the facts and begin the very unpleasant task of filing for unemployment benefits and looking for a new job.

That day I learned a lot about acceptance. Honestly, I had no other choice. The first thing I learned was to accept the present circumstances as they were. Someone once described it as having to stop barking and start biting. I had to do something about it, not just complain. This was a situation I had no control over preventing from happening. I couldn't run from it or fight it. Acceptance was my only choice.

It reminds me of the joke in which a woman calls a psychiatrist and says her husband thinks he is a chicken. The psychiatrist tells her to bring him in, and he'll cure the man. Later, the woman calls back, saying she's changed her mind. She'd rather keep her husband the way he is, saying, "Lord knows we can use the eggs."

When you find yourself in an unpleasant predicament, there is always the option to fight it. You can scream about what you've lost. Or you can accept it and try to put together something that is good. I've been told acceptance is riding the bus and facing the direction it is going.

Similarly, as an illness progresses to the point of being incurable, terminally ill patients may gradually become accepting of their situation. Maybe they feel they have lived a full life and fulfilled their purpose. Or, they are so sick and tired of being sick and just plain tired; they just want it to end. Maybe they can accept the terminal diagnosis intellectually but not emotionally.

Often it seems it is the family that is not accepting of the situation. One or more family members simply don't want to lose their loved one. This is a very normal, common-sense response. But the hard part comes when deep down inside as the family and their loved one understand there is no hope of recovery. They just can't bear to lose them. That is where real acceptance comes in. At some point, it becomes a matter of letting go and letting God. The hard part is knowing when.

When a serious illness develops and you are told that a cure isn't possible, you have a choice to fight on anyway or surrender to it. It is a very personal choice. Hospice does not discourage anyone from pursuing treatment.

Every hospice organization is always available to answer questions should you find yourself dealing with a medical crisis. Our primary purpose is to offer comfort, whether it be physical, spiritual, or emotional.

I have used the Serenity Prayer quite often in my life. It seems appropriate here: *God, grant me the serenity to accept the things I cannot change, the courage to change the things I can, and the wisdom to know the difference.*

Your Family Doctor

ONE OF THE many misconceptions or myths about hospice care is that you will lose the relationship you have with your family doctor should you choose to accept the service. In particular, one of the hesitations in calling hospice is the fear of having a new doctor with whom you are unfamiliar. We understand the fear, and, as with all aspects of hospice care, the recipient's concerns are listened to and addressed. With nearly every hospice, a plan is always worked out to which all involved agree. And the nice thing is that your wants are paramount when discussing who your physician will be. As a side note, your wants are paramount in your entire plan of care.

I was talking to a woman who had been the primary caregiver for her mother. She told me that she was on the verge of trying to find a specialist "who could refer her mother to the correct specialist," as she put it. My guess was that she might have arrived at the end of her rope.

Maybe you can relate to her? As the illness progresses up to the point of considering hospice, most patients have been visiting more and more specialists. Accordingly, a hospice doctor may be perceived as just one more specialist. By this time, after all of the many new medical people becoming involved, families just want to keep their own doctor.

If hospice is the choice, there are three options when it comes to deciding who the attending physician might be. First, you may retain your family doctor as your physician during this stage of your life. Your doctor, if comfortable with the situation, will then become a part of your extended hospice team and will consult with our hospice doctor regarding your care. Hospice understands that over a period of time, a person may develop a deep trust in his or her doctor. My mom was loyal to her family doctor to the very end. I, as well, trust my doctor above any other medical professional.

Even with the strong bond that sometimes exists between a patient and doctor, we have found that some physicians aren't comfortable with end-of-life issues. It is important to know that, yes, your family doctor knows you deeply; however, he or she may not have a competent understanding of the physical, emotional, and spiritual dynamics that are at play during the last stage of life. Even though your doctor may have no problem discussing treatments and procedures, he or she may find it almost impossible to discuss with you the reality of a terminal condition. That is human nature.

In the second scenario, your doctor may prefer not to be involved with your end-of-life care, but he or she may choose to continue addressing any other medical problems. Just as there are specialists in cardiology, digestive illnesses, cancer, etc., we are specialists in end-of-life care. And similar to your doctor working with other specialists, he or she may work with us in the same manner. The positive aspect of choosing a hospice doctor is having a doctor on your care team who will visit you where you live. Some general practitioners may not have that freedom.

Lastly, your doctor may decide not to be involved in your end-of-life care. This is a frequent and understandable occurrence. In this case, the family doctor relinquishes responsibility for your care, and the hospice's doctor will assume duties. Since care for someone in the last stage of life may require late-night decisions, having a hospice doctor assume full care makes sense. I might add, hospices still maintain contact with your family doctor regarding the progress of your illness and will notify him or her should changes in condition arise or death occur.

As with all situations involving patient care, hospice asks the question, "What does the person want?" There is no specific rule as to which of the scenarios to use. Hospice is here to help and will work out a care plan that satisfies the person who is ill while also keeping the family in mind. Hospice understands the importance of the doctor/patient relationship. You'll probably never meet a group in the medical field more eager to cater to your wants than those in hospice.

When you think about it, all through life you have been following your doctor's orders. If your situation in life begins to change, it may become very unsettling. Hospice will do everything to bring back a sense of normalcy. One of those ways is to offer the option of keeping someone close who understands you the most and who may be a lifelong friend, your family doctor.

The Life Business

Hospice is in the life business. Sounds like an oxymoron, but it is true. When setting up the initial consult with a family, hospice staff members will encourage as many family members to attend as wish to. One objective of this meeting is for the social worker to discuss important paperwork such as a living will.

Another objective, and an important part of this initial meeting, is for the social worker to inquire about the person's accomplishments, hobbies, and anything else that helps us really get to understand the individual. We know about the person's disease, but we now want to know about him or her as a person. Of special interest are family traditions and stories because these help us to develop a unique plan of care for the individual.

Many times during these conversations, the memories and the funny family stories of life come out. One daughter gave us insight by talking about her dad and his knack for turning the simplest event into a lifelong memory. For instance, one day during the first winter after she moved out west, the woman received an email from her dad. It simply said, "It snowed. I did the 'snow dance.' Love, Dad."

It was a family tradition that every year, during the first snowfall of the winter, the woman's dad would do the snow dance. He'd say that he was going outside and would take on the personality of a snowflake (use your imagination) and then do a ballet dance in the backyard. For years, during the first snowfall of the winter, the woman would call him to see if it was snowing in Ohio and if he had performed the snow dance.

In another instance, the son of a man being signed onto my hospice told how his father was Shampoo Man. Say what?

Shampoo Man? The son said that when he and his little brother were small, they did not like to have their hair shampooed. They would cry and fuss until the creation of Shampoo Man. After that time, they couldn't wait to have their hair washed. Their Dad would leave, and Shampoo Man would enter the room with his trusty cape that conveniently doubled as a towel. Laughing, the son also mentioned how his dad would press a sandwich down flat to "seal in the flavor."

As the father's life ebbed, the family gathered around his bedside, reminiscing. The father was able to hear about the legacy of memories and traditions that he had created. There was plenty of laughter that day, along with plenty of tears.

Not long ago, one of our social workers told me of a family whose grandmother was on our hospice. One granddaughter talked about the many opportunities that her grandmother had found to make wonderful memories. As the granddaughter talked, it was obvious that her grandmother had made a memory out of the mundane and a treasure out of a task. For instance, her grandmother had changed the name of a recipe on the side of a box of macaroni and cheese entitled "Rodeo Macaroni" to "Daddy-O-Macaroni."

For those families, their memories have lasted a lifetime. And it is those stories that help a family be of one frame of mind as they walk together into the next stage of a family member's life. At some point, these memories of life may be all that is left. They are the things that families will fight the hardest to keep.

Yes, hospice is in the life business. We help those on our service celebrate their lives. We are not talking about anything fancy. All you need is a gentle snowfall or a bottle of shampoo, or maybe a box of macaroni and cheese. It is such a good way to reminisce about life.

The Bitter End

"**M**AYBE WE SHOULD call hospice."
"Oh no, you don't! We're going to fight this to the bitter end!"

That was a scenario played out by an acquaintance of mine from church. He said he couldn't convince anyone in his family to call hospice and ask a few simple questions. Fighting the disease was perceived as being strong. They were trying to outsmart a disease that had no cure.

My question is, why? Why have a bitter end to your life? Life involves so many struggles, so why not enjoy the last stretch? Granted, it is difficult to determine when the last stretch has arrived. Hospice offers a pain-free life with your family at your side. The choice is always yours, but if medical science says there isn't a cure, why keep enduring painful treatments or experimental trials with their miserable side effects?

All of this activity will involve the ill person and a family member driving to wherever the treatment will take place. With most hospices, when you make the first call, we come to you to discuss your situation. It is hard to believe that one call is all you have to make. Plus, almost all hospices care for people where they live. No patients or family have to travel anywhere.

I don't want to die, but I have to accept the fact that I haven't heard of anyone currently on Earth who was born in the 1800s. They must've gone somewhere. Many have told me when they exhausted all treatment options and accepted their situation that they achieved a level of peace not experienced in quite a while.

If, and that's a big IF, people call hospice when they are months away from the life expectancy given by the doctor, they most likely will live longer than expected and be at home. Check the internet and see what you find regarding how hospice may improve life expectancy.

The reason for a longer life expectancy is simple. We stop attacking the body. We allow nature to follow its natural course. What we do is remove physical, emotional, and spiritual pain. As end-of-life care specialists, we know how to guide the family and patient through this stage. Studies by insurance companies have consistently shown people live longer under hospice care.

I was talking to Dr. Bob, a friend of mine. He said the general public's perception of hospice care is that it's a signal of giving up. In truth, that is a myth. Hospice doesn't give up on a person's life; rather, we help them embrace it. We celebrate life to the end.

CHAPTER 2
Experiencing Hospice

"The only certain measure of success is to render more and better service than is expected of you."

—Og Mandino

There Are No Dumb Questions

"THIS MAY BE a dumb question, but . . ." That preface to a question is something hospice staff frequently hear from family members of those on hospice. They might be asking about the illness, if there is more they can do to care for their loved one, or if they are "allowed" to do something in particular.

There are no dumb questions. We understand that families are under strain and sometimes aren't thinking as clearly as normal. To every question, we give an honest answer or reply with, "We'll see what we can do."

Since our care of the person and his or her family deals with all facets of life, the questions asked might not necessarily be of a medical nature. Often, the questions deal with last wishes. Surprisingly, questions regarding last wishes, or "bucket-list" type questions, most often deal with one-last-time desires. Many people on hospice want to do something one last time. My experience has been not many people want to "See Rock City" at the end of life.

Recently, Tammy, one of our nurses, completed arrangements to transport a man on service from his home to my hospice's in-patient facility, the Pickering House. The man was born and lived most of his life in rural Perry County. He and his son loved to fish together, and, as the years went by, his grandson joined them. After retirement, the man and his wife moved to Florida.

When the man became seriously ill, he and his wife moved back to their beloved Perry County to be cared for by his son- and daughter-in-law. Their plan was to stabilize the man's health so the family could go fishing at least once more. Regrettably, things didn't work out as planned, and the man was admitted to hospice.

Even though he was bedridden when we admitted him, the man wanted to remain at home. His wife and grown children cared for him there. In time, it became necessary for him to be brought to the Pickering House. His health was deteriorating, and additional nursing care could be administered there.

Arrangements were made, and the next morning the transport ambulance arrived. As the man was placed in the back of the ambulance, his wife joined him. She had the empty feeling that this was their last ride together. The man's son and teenage grandson were to follow in their car. Tammy had assisted the family in preparing him for the transfer and was to follow in her car.

But before everyone got in their respective cars, the son asked them to wait. Hesitantly, he asked Tammy, "This may be a dumb question, but . . . can we stop by the lake? It's on the way, and I'd like to take Dad fishing one more time."

"Sure!" was the quick reply from Tammy. As a hospice nurse, Tammy instinctively knew the importance of that question. Jubilant, the son exclaimed, "Dad, we're going fishing!"

Initially, the ambulance driver was stunned by the seeming absurdity of the question. However, remembering the many hours fishing with her dad while she was growing up helped her understand the importance of the request. This was not going to be just another patient transfer.

After the driver notified her dispatcher of the change in plans, the impromptu "fishing trip" began. A few miles outside of town, the entourage turned off US 22 and followed the narrow country road to Rush Creek Lake, the lake where the family had spent so many lazy days fishing. The slight sound of the gravel crunching and popping under tires broke the silence as the vehicles slowed to a stop in the parking area near the shore. I can't imagine what was going through each person's mind as they stared at the lake.

After a brief silence, the son asked, "Dad, do you want to try near the standing trees or fish off the dock?" Even though his dad was semi-comatose, the son knew his dad could hear. The son was painting a picture, reliving their many hours spent together fishing.

"Would you like to be near the water?" asked the driver.

Ever so carefully, she backed the vehicle toward the small boat dock. A tear blurred her vision as she realized that she was being allowed a small part in this intensely sacred event. Gingerly, everyone helped move the gurney onto the pier then stepped back. Words were not necessary. I've heard it said when a dad gives to his son, both laugh; when a son gives to his dad, both cry. There wasn't a dry eye.

"This looks like a good spot, Dad." Since childhood, how many times had he said those same words to his dad?

"You find a good place to sit down, Grandpa. I'll get the tackle box," said his grandson.

They were creating another day at the lake. The son then cupped his hands to bring up some lake water. As he let the lake water roll over his dad's hands, he could sense a smile on his face. It was obvious that the frustration his dad had experienced in his final months of not being able to go fishing was gone.

To those present, the entire universe boiled down to just that scene on the dock: Grandpa, son, grandson fishing. Observing this, the man's wife, almost whispering, said, "This will be forever in my heart. I will never forget this."

What started as a simple transfer from home to the Pickering House unfolded into an event that made a lifelong, life-changing impression on all of those involved. Tammy, the nurse, did not hesitate when the son asked if he could take his dad fishing one more time. She knew fishing didn't just mean fish. She sensed that fishing must've been an important part of this father/son relationship. It was just that simple.

The man was noncommunicative, but that didn't matter because men communicate through an activity more than they communicate by talking. This last fishing trip was a way for father and son to reminisce about their life together and to say a final goodbye. The man's son and grandson talked to him as if they were all fishing, but in reality they were communicating a lifetime of love and memories. Boys inherently follow their dads' example, not their advice. And what a profound example this was for the grandson.

Although losing a husband, a dad, a grandpa is sad, the family had good memories of the man's last day. Without realizing it, the son allowed the family's last hours together to be wonderful by doing something they had longed to do for a long time.

Hospice allows families to seize the moment to do what they feel is necessary to complete the life of their loved one and will try to assist if needed. Hospice doesn't change what is going to happen, but it changes *how* it is going to happen. And it may start with just a simple question.

Thy Will Be Done

It was difficult emotionally, but my wife Vickie and her sisters knew that at some point, they would become the caregivers for their big sister, Julie. For so long there had been hope that Julie's illness could be cured or at least controlled. But Julie had had enough. She said after more than a decade of fighting her disease, all she wanted was to be home. At her request, hospice was called.

Within hours of calling hospice, Julie was brought home from the hospital. Being on hospice service allowed Julie to be cared for in her home, in her own bed, and, of utmost importance, to be back in control of her life. Julie's three sisters mobilized to care for her.

Vickie knew that when it came to the point where Julie needed end-of-life care, she would do it; not a pleasant thought, but an easy decision. Yet, no matter how noble the intention, there is no way to prepare for such a situation. In too short of a time, everything seemed to change when the inevitable had to be accepted. Seeking inner strength, Vickie took a deep breath and prayed, "Thy will be done." It was a prayer she would repeat over and over during the next two weeks.

With the help of her other two sisters, Vickie tended to Julie in a way only a sister could. As Julie's condition deteriorated, Vickie would find herself softly repeating to herself, "Thy will be done" over and over. It gave her solace.

As the end seemed close, the thought occurred to Vickie to do something with Julie's hair. She knew Julie was going to Heaven but also knew Julie wouldn't want to go anywhere with "her hair looking like that." Lying in her bed, Julie was motionless, her breathing becoming much shallower and more intermittent. Experience told Vickie that her sister's hour was approaching, so Vickie decided not to disturb her.

The next morning brought a perfect fall day; clear skies and a gentle breeze. In late morning, while at the bedside of her deep-sleeping sister, Vickie said, "Julie, let's do something with your hair." She turned on a local Christian radio station and gathered everything needed. In a conversational voice, Vickie reminisced about their childhood with remember-the-time-we adventures as she shampooed Julie's hair, dried it, and brushed it the way Julie always liked it.

"That looks better," Vickie said. Leaning over, she whispered in Julie's ear, "There, you look good for Jesus. It's okay to go."

Within minutes, she noticed that Julie quit breathing. In the background, the song "Thy Will" by Hillary Scott was repeating the refrain "Thy will be done . . . Thy will be done." Julie was in His embrace.

Laying her head on Julie's shoulder, Vickie cried.

The end of life is a spiritual event and nothing else.

Fur Instead of Wings

As a woman walked through a dog shelter, she noticed a little black puppy in the back of one of the pens, shivering with fright. Without hesitation, she told the manager, "I'll take him." The woman said that for some reason, the little guy reminded her of a TV show she loved as a child. The show was about a private detective, Boston Blackie, who proclaimed himself as "a friend to those who have no friend." The woman, herself alone, said she immediately knew as soon as she saw the little black Labrador that the puppy would be her friend. The little puppy, which she named "Jeeves," did live up to her expectations as each gave the other companionship.

Regretfully, the one thing Jeeves couldn't do was protect his owner from disease. It wasn't long before the woman became ill. She succumbed to her illness within a year and died. Because the woman was alone with no family or friends, Jeeves was returned to the dog shelter, the same one where his life began. As luck would have it, the same shelter employee still worked there.

Soon after someone came to the shelter, looking for a pup. She was single, with only a sister living in the area. Even though she came into the shelter wanting a puppy, when she saw Jeeves sitting in the back of the pen, looking so sad, that was it. The manager told her of the young Lab's previous owner dying and how Jeeves had reminded that person of the TV show. She was a calm and pragmatic woman, saying, "Well, I guess this time I'll be the 'friend to the one who has no friend.'"

In no time, the two bonded. The woman, "Anne," led a busy life and would sometimes come home late, but Jeeves was always there. He listened attentively to her, whether she had a rough day or was happy following a good day. But ominous clouds began to gather a few years after she brought Jeeves home. Anne began to notice that she would tire easily. Other symptoms developed. Even though she was very successful and someone who fought and overcame many problems, this problem wouldn't surrender.

By now, the two had become inseparable, with Jeeves offering comfort as best he could while Anne's illness progressed. Over time, it came to the point where she faced an unpleasant decision. She either had to accept a bleak future of living in a facility and fighting an incurable disease or remain at home and make the call to hospice. For her, it was a relatively easy decision to make the call because the thought of giving up Jeeves was out of the question. That decision allowed Anne to be cared for at home with her beloved black Lab always at her side.

This event was brought to my attention while I was sitting in on one of our Interdisciplinary Team (IDT) meetings. During this weekly meeting, our staff meets to review each person on our hospice. Occasionally, a staff member brings up a situation that needs to be discussed.

Before bringing up Anne's plight at the meeting, her nurse and social worker had discussed several options concerning Jeeves' future. Having learned of his life story from the woman's sister, our nurse understood how important Jeeves was to Anne and, conversely, how important Anne was to Jeeves. But Anne could no longer live at her home. So, now what?

After a lively discussion in the IDT meeting, it was decided Jeeves would continue to live with Anne for as long as possible, whether in the Pickering House or somewhere else. Her nurse made arrangements to allow him to ride along in the ambulance with his best friend as she was brought to the Pickering House. Everyone attending the meeting hoped to meet Jeeves when he arrived.

Once Anne was in her room and settled in bed, Jeeves sat up at Anne's bedside and nudged his head under her hand. She painfully lifted her hand so he could push his head under it. He sat next to the bed with Anne's hand on his head as she slept. Making her first check on the two, the Pickering House nurse realized this arrangement wasn't going to work for very long.

In hospice, many of the problems faced do not deal with a disease or its symptoms. The problems deal with life. Most of the problems seem to be ones not found in medical books.

In short order, our staff came up with the idea to use what is called a bariatric bed. It is a bed used primarily for larger patients. Being wider than a normal bed, it would allow room for Jeeves to lie next to Anne without causing discomfort.

Soon, the woman was placed in the new bariatric bed, and Jeeves, with no encouragement needed, jumped on the bed and placed his head on her abdomen. Anne cried for joy when her companion snuggled next to her. She slowly lifted her hand and placed it on Jeeves' head. What a relief! And for a long time neither changed position, except when Jeeves needed to go outside for a few minutes.

Within a few days, comforted by Jeeves' around-the-clock presence, the woman peacefully left this world. Jeeves, however, wouldn't leave her side. After waiting until the funeral director arrived, and with a reverence only few would understand, Anne's nurse tenderly lifted the woman's hand off Jeeves, allowing the body to be removed. There were no words spoken and not a dry eye in the room.

When I talk to someone who has experienced hospice, what they remember primarily is how we met their emotional and spiritual needs. Rarely is the terminal condition ever mentioned. Every hospice staff member is immersed in giving care when there is no cure available. They are always thinking of the best way to offer comfort in a manner that benefits the person on hospice. Most importantly, it is done based on what the ill person *wants*, not necessarily according to what protocol is supposed to be followed in a certain situation.

Early on in our comforting Anne, she told her social worker how our staff's attention to Jeeves gave her peace of mind. The social worker assured her no matter the outcome, we would somehow care for her beloved black Labrador. And we did. After Anne's passing, our medical director brought Jeeves home with him to live on his rural property and run free with his other dogs.

This chain of events wasn't necessarily unusual in the hospice setting. Our care includes everyone affected by the illness, even if that "everyone" has four legs. In this case, it was a black Labrador named Jeeves. During his life, he demonstrated his gift by filling the emptiness of two people's lives.

Angels aren't always in heaven; they do their work on Earth. Some, as we learned from Jeeves, choose fur instead of wings.

A Wonderful Fall Wedding

IT'S BEEN SAID that death comes either too soon or too late. Society has been trying to make sure it doesn't come too soon. Fighting to the bitter end and doing whatever it takes to get one more day seems to be everyone's goal. But at what price? FAIRHOPE Hospice and Palliative Care, Inc. allows life to go on as normally as possible, like natural childbirth but on the other end of the spectrum. It is amazing—no, make that profound, what can happen when we allow life to just happen as it should.

In FAIRHOPE's case, we keep people in their home, wherever they call home, and active in life (as their health allows) even though the end may seem imminent. FAIRHOPE's purpose is to assist, not speed up or slow down the natural rhythm of life. The following story, which happened several years ago, is good to showcase how we focus on people's lives, not their illnesses.

Several years ago, in the spring, a young woman became engaged. What a joy for her mom! So many things to do! It was an exciting time as mom and daughter planned the wedding. The mom, "Jen," reminisced about when she was planning her own wedding with her mom. As June arrived, the plans were in full swing, and a fall wedding was in sight. However, by early July, the mom began tiring very easily. After several doctor visits, the mom broke the news to her daughter that she had Stage IV cancer. The cancer seemed to be growing rapidly, and the doctor estimated that the mother only had a few months of life remaining.

The daughter, understandably stunned, immediately decided to postpone her wedding to allow everyone to focus on her mother. She felt that her mom's situation was much more urgent and important than the wedding. Her mother absolutely refused to allow her to cancel the wedding, reasoning that while her life was coming to an end, her daughter's new married life was just beginning. Each woman wanted only to put the other first. The daughter eventually relented and kept the wedding date as planned.

The family knew of FAIRHOPE's compassion and opted to admit Jen onto hospice service. This allowed her to be cared for at home and still continue helping with the wedding preparations.

As the September days went by, Jen's pain level increased. Concern was growing that she would not be able to attend the wedding. Or worse, she might not live to see her daughter's important day. With less than ten days until the wedding, Jen was brought to the Pickering House, FAIRHOPE's hospice in-patient house, for one of its main purposes—symptom management. In this case, the symptom was pain. The Pickering House's staff carefully brought Jen's pain down to a tolerable level while keeping her fully aware of her surroundings; this was a very important key if she were to watch her little girl walk down the aisle.

Probably the most important duty of a mother on her daughter's wedding day is to be nearby when needed. And Jen was determined to be just that for her daughter. In preparation, Jen's home nurse, Katie, spent the night before the wedding at the family's home. The next morning, Katie accompanied Jen to the event, even going as far as assisting with getting Jen ready. Everyone could now focus on the special wedding day, knowing that medical assistance was nearby to help. Katie would be there on hand, sitting with the congregation during the wedding.

As the "Wedding March" began, all eyes turned toward the back. The guests were startled to see three people begin the walk down the aisle. With sniffles accompanying the music, Jen was escorted on one side by her daughter, the bride, and on the other side by the bride's brother. I think that even the church mouse had a tear in his eye as the three slowly approached the altar. Jen had done it!

Katie sat with Jen during the ceremony. Jen being able to watch her daughter profess her vows was vital to her. The wedding reception, even though it was held in the church building, was not as important to Jen. She said the celebrating was for her daughter. Jen was brought into a separate room in the church, converted into a small, quiet area by Katie, where Jen could lie down. There she rested and spoke to Katie about needing to talk to her dad, who was already in heaven. Katie knew by this small comment that Jen was preparing for her transition into the next dimension of life, and she was also preparing her family.

Jen was brought back to the Pickering House later in the day, exhausted but at peace. She had achieved her ultimate goal of watching her little girl get married.

This had been a truly special day for everyone, even the wedding photographer, who went way beyond what anyone expected and worked through the weekend preparing all of the photos. On Monday, with her family around her bed, Jen reviewed the wedding and reception pictures. On Wednesday, she would breathe her final breath and go to be with her dad.

The last stage of life is meant to be lived to its fullest. With the assistance of FAIRHOPE's staff, who truly understand that life is measured more by depth than length, this, too, can be accomplished by those at the end of life. Mother and daughter proved just that.

The end of life is not always as much about medical knowledge as it is about finding your purpose and fulfilling it with those you love. FAIRHOPE Hospice, as do many hospices, focuses on the life business. We allow life to go on as it should, adjusting plans as needed and including an assist for a wonderful fall wedding.

An Order of Fried Chicken

In late October, a man accepted FAIRHOPE Hospice and Palliative Care's compassionate care. Prior to signing onto our hospice, he had been a patient at a Columbus area hospital. When he was admitted to FAIRHOPE's in-patient hospice facility, the Pickering House, on October 31, he definitely had an attitude. The man was to be our guest for a few days for a respite stay. One of the main reasons for the attitude was his complaint about what he considered to be not very good treatment given to him at the hospital. He said no one had listened to him, nor had they seemed to care.

One of the little things that bugged the man about his stay at the Columbus hospital was that he couldn't have what he really wanted to eat for dinner. He was told that based upon his illness and what was "good for him," he was limited to only two choices of food that he could order.

This reminds me of the humorous story of a passenger on a transatlantic flight. The flight attendant asks each passenger if they want dinner. She asks one particular passenger if he'd like dinner.

"What are my choices?" he asks.

"Yes or no," is the reply.

Evidently, this person arriving at the Pickering House was expecting more of the same from us. He quickly learned FAIRHOPE, as with any hospice, wouldn't be more of the same.

Not long after the man's arrival, a Pickering House STNA, Carla, came into his room to introduce herself. It didn't take her long to realize he was agitated. "Well, what can we do for you that would make you feel better?" Carla inquired. The man said it was something we couldn't help him with because the only thing that would make him feel better was fried chicken from his favorite restaurant. "Which one?" she asked.

"Dodson's" was the reply.

Before I go too far, what was "typical FAIRHOPE" in Carla's inquiry was that she was already thinking perhaps something could be done to get to the root of the man's agitation. With a tepid sigh, he said he was from New Lexington, Ohio, and his favorite restaurant was Dodson's on Broadway. He mentioned how he liked everything at Dodson's, with the fried chicken being his favorite. He always had French fries to go with it.

Carla sympathized with him because she, too, loved Dodson's chicken. She also knew that he wasn't just missing fried chicken. Since he had mentioned a particular restaurant, she knew that this was a vitally important one-last-time type of request in disguise. Leaving the man's room, Carla thought maybe one day during his respite stay she would bring him some Dodson's chicken. Since Carla lives in the New Lexington area, she planned to bring in some the next day.

However, Carla's background in hospice care told her that in this stage of life, things might change in a hurry. It was imperative that the time to make the man's wish a reality was now. Regretfully, it was a busy night, and the forty-mile round trip to Dodson's would take her too long.

The idea crossed her mind that her daughter might be able to help and bring in the food that night. It happened to be Halloween night, and there was the possibility her daughter wouldn't be available. By the grace of God, her daughter was home and willing to help. Carla called Dodson's and ordered the chicken for carry-out. She made arrangements with her daughter to pick up the order and bring it to the Pickering House.

When a situation like this arises at FAIRHOPE Hospice, our

employees rise up to meet it. So, while the chicken was on the way, our cook, Linda, said she would wait until Carla's daughter arrived with the order of fried chicken before she put the fries in the fryer. That way they would be fresh and warm. Once the fried chicken arrived, it was warmed up a bit in the oven while the fries were made.

When the meal was brought into the man's room, he was stunned. Then he did something he hadn't done in a long time. His bottom lip began to quiver, and he started to cry. His meal was brought in with the chicken still in the very familiar Dodson's box. Memories flooded in. Through his tears, the man thanked Carla.

His family thought Carla was being facetious when they were told the chicken was freshly delivered from Dodson's. Once it sank in as to the amount of energy put into fulfilling the request, they were speechless, and there were more tears. The family just could not believe the effort put into what appeared to be a trivial comment.

I honestly don't think the man was that hungry for something to eat. In the last stage of life, the need and desire for food goes away. And in that vein, any hunger at the end of life does not necessarily indicate a desire for food but a longing to complete one's life. This man was fortunate enough to have a hunger that the employees of FAIRHOPE Hospice understood.

The importance of eating his favorite meal, Dodson's modest fried chicken and French fries, satisfied the man's desire to taste a favorite indulgence one last time. He was able to relive one of the enjoyable parts of his life. More importantly, it satisfied his longing to be accepted as a normal person again. It fulfilled his longing to have the autonomy to ask for something and receive it. Through that one gesture of simply ordering a meal, Carla satisfied his hunger, acknowledged his longing, and helped return him to some sense of who he had been before his illness.

The most important part of FAIRHOPE Hospice's care is listening. When someone has entered the last stage of life, casual comments are not just casual comments. What ill people bring up in conversation is what is vital for them to complete their life, even if it seems insignificant . . . as insignificant as an order of fried chicken.

Basic Nursing

Nursing is one of those careers that has steadily evolved. As the field expands and adds more responsibilities, what that career actually entails seems to be getting less clear-cut. I think the simplest definition of a nurse is "a person trained to care for the sick and infirm." On the other side of the coin, the American Nursing Association states, "Nursing is the protection, promotion, and optimization of health and abilities, prevention of illness and injury, alleviation of suffering through diagnosis and treatment of human response, and advocacy in the care of individuals, families, communities, and populations."[1]

Not too long ago the hospice where I work received a thank-you card from a man whose wife had died on our service. In the card, the man thanked "the nurse who sat on the floor at (my wife's) bedside with us when she had expired. (Our nurse) Tammy waited patiently and lifted our spirits while waiting for the funeral director to arrive to retrieve the body."

The man's wife had died at home in her bedroom. Since no one wanted to leave her alone, they sat on the floor. Tammy knew the family needed comfort, so she, too, sat on the floor with them. I've heard it said, "People don't care how much you know until they know how much you care." Tammy cared enough to take as long as was necessary to wait for the funeral director's arrival. That simple gesture meant so much to the deceased's family.

---

1 American Nurses Association[36] (36) ANA Considering Nursing... Retrieved Dec 2018 (ANA website 2015)... found at **acadamia.edu** on 7/17/2020 and in Wikipedia

Absolutely, there is a need for advanced-degree nurses, nursing professors, directors, leaders, etc. But at the end of life, the only need is for "a person trained to care for the sick and the infirmed," a hospice nurse.

Holding Hands

Hospice is as much a family-oriented organization as it is a person-focused organization. The obvious reason being when a family member is terminally ill, the whole family is affected. As such, hospice is alert to the needs of the family. We offer a calming presence to reduce any additional disruption to the nerve-wracking situation of caring for a terminally ill family member.

What I find so gratifying about being a part of the hospice philosophy of care is that when somebody throws us a curveball, we respond; we don't react. A good example of how we respond occurred a few years ago. Initially, it looked to be fairly straightforward. A man was admitted on our hospice, and we provided care for him at his home with his wife as his primary caregiver.

As the weeks went by, the wife herself developed a medical condition that required minor surgery. While recuperating, she was not going to be able to give her husband the attention he needed. Both were distraught because to be separated when they needed each other so desperately was unfathomable. The situation was brought up in our Interdisciplinary Team (IDT) meeting to get input from all of the staff. Everyone discussed the situation and what would be the best option of how to solve the dilemma. Notice that I said "how" to solve, not "if" it could be solved.

This was one of the many predicaments that fall into the "Now what?" category. The solution turned out to be quite simple. While needing a few days to recuperate, the wife wouldn't be able to care for the love of her life, so he was brought to the Pickering House. Since the woman only needed a couple of days to recuperate, our social worker arranged for her to stay overnight with her husband at the Pickering House in his room. When she arrived, her husband reached out for her. That evening they held hands until they went to sleep.

Hospice knows there is a solution to any dilemma. It may be as basic as helping a couple be together, stay connected, and just hold hands.

Not a Medical Event

June is the month for weddings, and an integral part are the heartfelt vows. In hospice, we get to know the people on service and their families very well. Sometimes we are blessed to see the wedding vows fulfilled. On one consecrated evening, several of our staff were able to witness the final vow in its most elemental form.

The wife was in the Pickering House for end-of-life care. During her stay, her nurse had noticed the patient's husband of over fifty years never left her bedside. On this particular evening when the nurse entered the patient's room, her experience told her that their final wedding vow, "'til death do us part," was about to be fulfilled.

Seeing the unflinching devotion of the husband, the nurse knew exactly what had to be done. With the help of Pickering House aides and housekeeping staff, they helped the husband get into bed to lie with his actively dying wife. Although she had previously not responded to any stimuli, as he lay down with her and wrapped his arms around her, her facial expression softened, her body relaxed, and her breathing calmed. The husband held her so close; she knew she was once again in his arms.

No medication could ever bring that kind of comfort and peace. It was so beautiful and heart-wrenching at the same time. During this entire event no words were spoken; the silence was golden.

The end of life is a sacred experience; it is not a medical event. Hospice understands.

Where's the Other Sock?

One of the words you don't hear too often when talking about hospice care is "laundry." Yep, good old-fashioned bath towels and dirty socks. I bring the subject up because about ten years ago, I received a phone call from the volunteer coordinator, asking if I knew how to do laundry. I asked her if she had thought of hiring a maid. In a dry voice, she informed me that the spouse of someone on service had back issues and couldn't get down the stairs to the basement, where the washer and dryer were. The husband, on our service, used to do that chore, but he couldn't anymore. The dirty clothes were piling up.

As a patient-contact volunteer, my purpose is to help those on our service continue to lead as normal a life as possible. And nothing falls into the normal life category better than dirty clothes. I accepted the assignment. Within a few visits, the routine developed that I would stop by the house on Tuesday morning, take the clothes the wife had sorted and go downstairs, wash them, and dry them. Since it was just the two of them, there weren't that many loads to be done. After I brought the clothes back upstairs, the three of us would fold them while watching *The Price is Right*.

Eventually, the woman told me how to get stains out of polyester. I showed them how to fold fitted sheets, and the husband explained how he mated all of the socks. It is amazing how people can bond while folding clothes.

The philosophy of hospice care centers on continuing to live life, not preventing death. A part of living a normal life is continuing to do the normal mundane activities of life, such as laundry. And yes, we seemed to always finish one sock short.

Mom's Favorite Color

MANY OF THE articles I write are from my own experiences as a patient-contact volunteer, and some are the result of what I hear from our staff. However, I find it a little difficult to obtain information from our staff, be it those who visit people where they live or those who work in our in-patient facility, the Pickering House. The main reason, I feel, is that they see nothing momentous in what they do. Yes, they are totally committed to those on our service, but they look at it as simply, "If they need help, I'll help." And true help is often the result of intuition.

Those I work with are immersed in hospice, not just employees. We instinctively know that when we hear a whimsical statement at the end of life, those statements are, in reality, one-last-time laments. Whenever I converse with people who have experienced our indefinable compassion, they always mention something we did that would seem mundane. Yet, those things are always what people remember.

For example, a woman mentioned that one of our STNAs did her mom's nails "in Mom's favorite color" only days before her passing. Doing her mom's nails was the only thing mentioned specifically when praising our service. Yes, she complimented us on our attentiveness and compassion. However, her mom's nails being tended to was, above all else, the only act specifically mentioned.

I think that an important reason hospice has a positive effect on people during their time of unthinkable crisis is because we focus not on just little things, but the little things that matter.

Nothing is Insignificant

Most advertisements I've seen for a medical practice or medical facility of any type talk about how caring, and of course, how compassionate they are. But they never tell you exactly what they do to define what makes them caring or compassionate. Maybe acts of compassion are considered insignificant. When you are a patient at any type of medical facility or medical practice that emphasizes how caring it is, the focus quickly changes from you to your illness when one of the staff says, "Okay, let's have a look."

I was talking to a woman whose mother had been on hospice. She mentioned that she had never forgotten how tenderly the Pickering House STNA would touch her mother. The woman said that even if just brushing her mother's hair, the STNA would first gently touch her mother's arm as if she was touching velvet. "She was so empathetic, so caring," the woman wistfully said. Even though her mother had died several years ago, the woman's eyes started to moisten as we spoke. "The hospice STNA's empathy touched me so deeply."

Of all that happened while her mother was ill, the tender way in which the hospice STNA physically touched her mother was one of the first things she mentioned. It is interesting that when I am talking to someone familiar with a person who was on hospice, he or she rarely mentions the illness or disease. But the illness generally dominates the conversation if a person died elsewhere outside of hospice, fighting it to the bitter end.

I think that is because everyone in hospice, especially the nurse's aides and STNAs, knows that in the last weeks of life, nothing is insignificant.

The Importance of Place

ONE OF THE misconceptions, or myths, of hospice is that it is a place, some sort of medical building, the notion being if you sign onto hospice care, you will have to go somewhere. In fact, you stay where you live, whether it is your home, a family member's home, a friend's home, a nursing home, or an assisted living community.

However, not to muddy the waters, but there are some hospices in America that do operate care facilities for their patients. When the famous *Washington Post* columnist Art Buchwald admitted himself into a Washington DC area hospice, he moved into the facility. That particular hospice didn't visit patients in their homes as most hospices do. Most hospice facilities offer in-patient and short-term respite care.

When a hospice cares for people who live in their house, hospice personnel understand that it is the patient's home and not theirs. Therefore, the person may have the bed set up wherever he or she wishes. As a patient-contact volunteer, several of my patients preferred to sleep in their living room recliners because they were more comfortable. It was *their* home, after all. So that was where they slept.

In your home, the feeling of being in control is brought back to you. In a hospital, you lose the feeling of being in charge. The same holds true in any type of institution. At home, you are in charge, and during this stage of your life, being in charge is one of the most important aspects of life.

Hospice recognizes the importance of place.

Our Bedside Staff

There is normally no obvious doorway opening to signal when the last stage of life has been entered. But when ill people feel they have had enough, and they no longer want to focus on "fighting it," that is when hospice should be called. In almost every discussion I've had with surviving family members, I will hear something to the effect, "If only I knew how supportive and reassuring everyone would be, I would have called sooner."

My opinion of why I hear that particular comment so often is due to the sensitivity of our team, referred to as "the bedside staff." They include RNs, LPNs, STNAs, social workers, and chaplains. I often hear people ask in so many words, "Where did you find such an approachable, compassionate group?"

One lesson I have learned from working in hospice is that what we do is not usually a high-tech skill. It's just down-to-earth listening to what terminally ill people need and serving those needs. Listening is at the core of the compliments that we receive. Our social workers compassionately listen to what terminally ill people desire, then assist them in obtaining it. Many times what is wanted is to do something one final time. I have witnessed and been blessed to be a part of occasions when our staff assisted in making a one-last-time wish come true.

Every week, my hospice has an Interdisciplinary Team meeting, otherwise known as our "team" meeting. The purpose of this is for our medical staff, social services, management, and other employees to gather and discuss each of those on our hospice. During the team meeting, thank-you cards received during the past week are passed around for each staff member to read. When reading the cards, what strikes me is that during such a high-stress time for a family, they invariably mention the littlest things. Everything mentioned seems so incidental, almost not worth mentioning until you understand the context in which it took place.

Most of these little kindnesses mentioned are carried out by our bedside staff. Not only do they listen, but they act upon what the person is talking about. In one of the cards was written, "We have never experienced anything like your service." The writer continued on to share that every person he and his family met on our staff exceeded their expectations. "Every one of them," he repeated.

Hospice is a good choice when the unthinkable may be on the horizon. To someone unfamiliar with hospice, what may not be obvious is that we are as much a spiritual, emotional, and people-oriented organization as we are a medical one, maybe more so.

Our bedside staff understands that the people they are caring for are going through a time they knew would come, but so soon? We listen to terminally ill people's concerns, and their families' as well, in order to find out what their hopes and fears are so we can base our plan of care on what information they give us. The nurses take all the time necessary to clarify information or instructions in care a family may not have understood. With shared understanding, the bedside staff gently guides all involved through the end-of-life process.

Many families have told me how important it was that, when they were expressing their concerns, our bedside staff listened to them while not interrupting the conversation. They compassionately listened. When I was at our booth during the annual county fair, a person stopped by and told me what impressed him about what hospice did for his family was, "Your chaplain listened. He let me talk. He sat down next to me and let me tell him what I was afraid of." He thought for a minute and added, "I realized later that the chaplain has probably heard the same story many times, but he sat there and listened. God bless him, he listened."

Isn't that thought-provoking? With all the experience and knowledge our chaplain possessed, what really stood out for this man was the fact that we listened.

On the medical side, the families tend to look to our nurses as the leading experts on pain and symptom management. Yet, what families tell me is how important it was for our nurse aides and nurses to teach them how to simply care for and comfort their loved ones. Whenever people tell me about their experience with hospice, what invariably comes through is the empathy they felt when discussing something with any of our bedside staff. One man told me that the minute the nurse aide came in the front door, he knew she would take care of his mom. He told me of how he felt completely at ease and knew that his whole family was now in good hands.

In the last days or months of life, medical knowledge is no longer important. What becomes of paramount importance to ill people is that they arrive at the end of life on their terms and no one else's. That is what we try to do, and that is probably the hardest aspect for families and the curative medical profession to understand.

People may want to focus their remaining time on sharing memories, passing on family stories, and imparting the wisdom they have learned. They may give remembrances or mementos to someone special in their life. They may wish to settle disputes with people or make peace with God. And our mothers most especially just want to make sure that no matter how old their children are, they will be okay.

I sat at my mother's bedside during her last hours and told her that she had done a wonderful job raising me. I reassured her I would be okay. I thought she was in a coma, but she faintly, unmistakably, smiled.

When in a conversation about where I work, people often

tell me they are too emotional to work in hospice. In reality, emotion is one of the traits most sought during the interview process of a candidate for our bedside staff. Those who have experienced hospice often bring up how the staff with whom they had contact empathetically listened.

Truly great moments can be beautifully wrapped in what others may consider a small one. A moment that is only understood by the bedside staff of RNs, LPNs, STNAs, chaplains, and social workers.

Beyond the Person in the Bed

ONE DISTINCTION THAT makes hospice care different from other areas of medicine is the Medicare requirement for volunteer involvement. Volunteers must provide some of the day-to-day administrative and/or direct patient-contact services. In fact, it is specified that the total of the volunteers' efforts must be in an amount that, at a minimum, equals 5 percent of the total patient-care hours of all paid hospice employees and contract staff. Therefore, volunteers aren't just a nice idea; they are a requirement.

The idea behind requiring volunteers to be a part of hospice is to foster a feeling of normalcy and companionship with the person being cared for. In other words, the volunteers' presence as members of the hospice team helps to remove some of the sterile atmosphere of medical care. Their role is one of compassionate service. I doubt many people think about the importance of a hospice volunteer when they call us for help.

Our volunteers ingrain a feeling of balance into our hospice care that is not found anywhere else in the realm of medical care. That dimension of hospice is one of the items that tend to catch people off guard once they have agreed to our compassionate help. The wife of a man on service told me that as her husband was fighting his disease over a lengthy period, he had nine surgeries, which included "surrendering a few organs" and chemotherapy. Plus, he endured at least a dozen external radiation treatments.

As an afterthought, the woman added, "He got through with the help of quite a few pills and patches." She said everything became a blur. She just wanted to go back to the way it was.

But then she commented, "When I called hospice, you let me stop being a caretaker and become his wife again. Thank you."

Once the woman's husband was admitted to hospice, a calmness settled over both her and her husband. The nurse suggested having a volunteer visit once a week to allow the wife to take a break for a few hours. She agreed, and a schedule was decided upon for a hospice volunteer to come to her home once a week. As it turned out, when the volunteer arrived, he would sit, talk, and "mainly listen" to her for several hours. Hours in which the wife had planned to run her weekly errands to get groceries, etc. She laughed as she told me she never did go grocery shopping and would always end up calling her son the next day to shop for her. "He never did use the coupons I gave him."

After all she had endured while her husband was so ill, what the woman remembered most was how the volunteer seemed to understand her situation. "I never thought that I needed a volunteer, but the social worker was right." She said her volunteer had no agenda other than to bring some routine back into her life.

The area of volunteering I am talking about is patient contact. Patient-contact volunteers are in a position to connect deeply with people on service, as well as with their families, providing the home-care team with insights as to the impact of care being provided. The patient-contact volunteer may become a liaison between people receiving care, their families, and the home-care team.

Often, people will tell me they want to become hospice volunteers, but they don't like the idea of being with someone who is seriously ill when no one else is there to assist. Should you want to volunteer, there is an almost limitless list of possibilities for what you can do. Many opportunities do not involve contact with a hospice patient or the patient's family.

As a volunteer, you choose in what area you'd like to be involved. You may want to help with fundraisers or help make lap blankets for those on hospice. Some hospices need veterans to visit with fellow veterans. In many hospices, volunteers bring their talents and help in areas not explored before.

Fellow volunteers have told me that it seems most of what they do is so mundane, so unimportant. In actuality, what volunteers do is ordinary. Our volunteers are ordinary people doing very simple, ordinary work. My own experience has been that what we do in end-of-life care is definitely noticed. The duties may seem unimportant and, as I've heard it described, colorless. They are not. The many thank-you cards we receive and the conversations I have had with the general public tell me that what both our patient-contact and non-contact volunteers do is profound. And it seems like most actions that the volunteers view as insignificant were the ones that the family saw as profound. There is such an importance to just being there.

The relationship between the hospice family and the patient-contact volunteer can be deep. For example, after one of the people I accepted as a volunteer assignment died, my volunteer manager notified me. I knew this was a very private family. My manager told me they were going to have a family-only memorial service at a later date. I was saddened because there wouldn't be a funeral, allowing me to talk to the spouse and extended family. I was not surprised because I knew the family and understood their wish for this special time for their family to gather together.

About a month later, the man's wife called me and invited me to the service. I was the only person attending who was not an immediate family member. Because of my involvement during the time of intense crisis, I had been more or less "adopted" and became a part of the family. That experience made me realize the importance of patient-contact volunteers.

Each hospice has its own training program, so volunteers are well prepared for what they will experience. Our training program is comprehensive and, believe it or not, enjoyable and motivating.

Hospice volunteers help to put the person back in the patient and bring a sense of normalcy to a family. Their presence helps all involved to focus on their loved ones and push the illness aside. Their reach extends and makes an impact well beyond the person in the bed.

All You Have to Do Is Ask

When I was very young, Mom would not allow me to drink a full bottle of pop. So she'd pour a glass for me, then stick a stopper in the neck of the bottle of pop. She said that plugging the bottle would keep the drink from going flat. Meaning that it would lose its "fizz" caused by carbonation.

What made me think of that was a woman who was recently staying at my hospice's in-patient facility, the Pickering House. She asked one of our STNAs, Carla, if she could have a Dr. Pepper. Since the carbonation in it would cause her to have hiccups, she asked if she could have a "flat Dr. Pepper."

No matter what those on our service request, our staff will do what they can to fulfill it. In this instance, it would take at least twenty-four hours for an opened Dr. Pepper to go flat. After thinking about it, Carla opened a can of Dr. Pepper and poured it into a glass with the plan to let it sit for a while. She knew it would eventually lose its carbonation and hence go flat.

As Carla was ready to put the can in the recycling container, an idea came to her: "If she wants a flat Dr. Pepper, I'll give her a flat Dr. Pepper." She took the can outside and stepped on it to flatten it. She washed it, then put it on a paper towel and took it to the lady's room. "I've got your flat Dr. Pepper," she said with pride.

The woman was startled at first but then burst into laughter. FAIRHOPE's STNAs know that laughter often makes the best medicine to heal a lot of hurts. We do whatever we can to heal those hurts, even if it falls a little flat. All you have to do is ask.

Custard from Heaven

The Pickering House's cook, Linda, was visiting the room of a person on our hospice as he talked about breakfast options. A few family members were also present, and the discussion was lively. Talking about food at the end of life always conjures up family memories.

When someone is admitted for a few days, Linda sits down and talks to the person and his or her family. She learns about the individual's favorite food and how he or she likes it prepared. Linda is never in a hurry when talking to someone on service or the person's family about food; people's preferences are so important.

In this instance, she learned the man on service loved the custard-filled doughnuts from Donut World. He lamented that he wasn't able to chew food anymore. His diet had been relegated to soft foods, such as Jell-O, scrambled eggs, and soup.

Understanding his sadness at the loss of one of his favorite foods, Linda knew there had to be something she could do. She also guessed that if he mentioned the custard doughnut, then he must like the custard in particular. After she left the man's room, on a whim she called Donut World and asked if she could purchase a cup of custard. The answer was a quick "Sure!"

Linda said she would come right over. The person who answered the phone had no idea who Linda was, or that she was on duty at the Pickering House. As she left, Linda told the charge nurse she would be back shortly.

When Linda arrived at Donut World, the person at the counter asked why she needed just a cup of custard. Linda explained the Pickering House had someone staying for a few days, and his favorite doughnut was the custard doughnut from their shop. Since the man's disease had progressed to the point where it was no longer safe for him to chew or digest solid food anymore, he was resigned to the fact that he'd never again enjoy his favorite doughnut. This revelation caused the cashier to pause for a moment with a blank stare. She couldn't believe that anyone would think to make such an effort, let alone actually come over to buy just a cup of custard.

Thinking back on this simple conversation, I believe most people would have empathized with the man on service, agreeing it certainly was too bad he couldn't have the custard doughnut. Linda is a first-class baker. She could easily have just made some custard. But, Linda is an employee of FAIRHOPE Hospice and Palliative Care. We don't think that way.

The person was in the last stage of life, and he craved something in particular. During this stage, what seems like idle yearning can be a deep-down wish. So many people, when they finally sign onto our service, have been told for a very long time that they couldn't eat this or eat that as they wanted. At hospice, you may still receive what you wish for, even if it can't be eaten.

In this particular situation, the man wanted a custard doughnut from a specific place. Since he mentioned the name of the doughnut shop, Linda knew that was of importance. Attention to the little details is what makes her and all of the staff such a wonderful group. They listen to the people under our care.

When Linda returned with that cup of custard, the man's family was curious to know what it was. At first, they couldn't believe she would go to such an effort for a seemingly trivial desire, and all she brought back was a regular cup of custard at that. Regular? As the man's wife slowly fed him a spoonful of the custard, he savored the taste and said, "Ah, custard from heaven."

Over one hundred years ago, playwright Henrik Ibsen said, "A thousand words will not leave so deep an impression as one deed." What an impact we can make at the end of one's life with one simple act of kindness and understanding! *Doughnut* let us forget this!

Peanut Butter and Banana Sandwich, Coming Up

EVER NOTICE HOW important food is? I imagine helping you to stay alive is fairly high on everyone's importance-of-food list. But as an illness progresses, a person's interest in food might wane. Sometimes the illness dictates that certain foods may not be eaten anymore. Many of those who contact hospice have been restricted as to what they can eat, maybe because of the reaction certain drugs have with food or perhaps the illness has caused digestive problems. The fact is, as a disease becomes more intrusive, eating is progressively more restricted. Through it all, the ill person and caregiver have little, if any, control over the situation.

One of the subtleties of hospice compassion is how we put the ill person, as much as possible, back in control of his or her life. By this stage of life, food's importance in sustaining physical health has now been replaced by food's importance in sustaining emotional health. One segment of emotional health involves having the control to make decisions. Another segment of emotional health is being able to ask and receive what you wish for most.

After a lengthy period of diet restrictions, how nice it must be to order and receive whatever you want to eat, whether it can be eaten or not. The request for food may be for a treat, such as a Dilly Bar from Dairy Queen, or it may be a favorite meal from a restaurant. The hospice where I work recently brought someone at the Pickering House their favorite meal. It was a T-Bone steak from the person's lifelong favorite restaurant.

As part of the hospice philosophy of care, we believe it is paramount that at the end of life, the control to ask and receive is yours. Fulfilling wishes for a favorite food is one way we do it. Had Elvis been on our service, I'll bet there would've been one peanut butter and banana sandwich comin' up.

Chester, Our Cat

The Pickering House is my hospice's in-patient facility. Many visitors don't know that we have a resident cat, Chester, at the Pickering House. That is just fine with him. I might point out that since the first day it was opened, the Pickering House has been meticulously cleaned daily to protect anyone with animal allergies. If someone who has a cat allergy is staying there, we keep the person's door closed.

When Chester was still "new in these parts," a woman was admitted to the Pickering House for end-of-life care. Arriving at the Pickering House, her daughter followed as the nurse and aide accompanied the transport ambulance attendants guiding the gurney into her room. Chester quietly followed the entourage into the room and lay down at the daughter's feet. A fast friendship developed.

During this stage of life, the illness is not the problem. The problem may be relationships, whether with family or with God. In this case, the mother and daughter had a few issues to work out, and heartfelt discussions took place in the room. Chester was always at the daughter's feet.

Several days after her arrival, the mother died. The daughter, of course, was upset and went to the Pickering House's chapel to be alone. As she was slumped in a chair, crying, Chester, who had followed her, jumped onto her lap and began to meow softly. For almost an hour as the initial emotion ran its course, Chester held on, resting his head on the woman's stomach and softly meowing.

That was the first time any of our staff saw Chester console anyone, but it is a scenario that is now seen more frequently. Chester demonstrated very soon after his arrival he wasn't just another pretty fluff of fur but one of our compassionate staff.

The primary purpose of hospice is comfort care. That care is administered in whatever way is appropriate by anyone on our staff, even by Chester, our cat.

Pets are Included

THERE ARE MANY areas we can address when talking about our health and wellness. And no matter what illness or problem we are talking about, if you have a pet, it is affected. The home-side staff of hospice deals with all sorts of pets, ranging from the usual dogs and cats to hamsters, cockatiels, parrots, and fish. Although, to be honest, I've never met a fish that had more than a passing interest in what was going on.

In discussions of serious illness or personal dilemma, the focus is naturally on the patient receiving the care and attention, not the pet. As in the arena of curative medicine, hospice directs attention toward the person on service, but rarely is that our only focus. What makes hospice unique is that we offer our assistance to anyone affected by the terminal diagnosis. Those who receive attention may include immediate family, extended family, friends, neighbors, and even pets. Pets? Say, what?! Yes, even pets.

Should someone still residing in his or her home sign onto hospice, the whole routine of life will be disrupted, sometimes a little bit and sometimes substantially. A team of personnel, including an STNA, nurse, social worker, spiritual care coordinator or chaplain, volunteer, and doctor is assigned to the family. At one time or another, most of the team members will visit at least once with the family. This activity may disrupt the family routine. Sensing that something is wrong with their owner, coupled with the change in the old routine, can upset pets.

When visiting someone still living at home, many of the staff keep dog treats and cat treats with them. This shows how family and pets are noticed and included in our care of the family. It is another subtle way that illustrates how hospice care is different. One of the people I would visit as a volunteer had two Siamese cats. I'm not saying they were unfriendly, but they didn't like anyone, including their owners. On my visits I always brought cat treats and placed them in the entrance foyer. By the end of two months of weekly visits, the cats would rub against me as I sat by their owner's bedside. I guess I felt special that they finally included me.

As an example of how much we understand their importance to the family, pets are allowed to stay overnight should their owners need to spend time at the Pickering House, my hospice's in-patient facility. By doing so, we make sure pets are not left alone. Having their faithful companions stay with them is comforting to both the people who are on service and their families.

Pets, as they always seem to do, can also help to bring a little levity into what is a somber situation. In another scenario as a patient-contact volunteer, I accepted an assignment of a family who had a schnauzer named Shultz. As was my norm, I gave their dog a Beggin' Strip doggy treat when I came for the first visit. It didn't take Shultz long to figure out that when I came, he was going to get a treat. The father of "Jimmy," the person on service, said, "I can always tell when you're way down the road because about when you are due, Shultz sits on the back of the couch, watching. As soon as he sees you, he runs through the house barking, then jumps back on the couch, then back through the house."

Dogs are very intuitive and have a sense of who is good and who isn't. I would visit a family with a dachshund named Oscar (as I think most of them are). Two things were interesting about Oscar. The first was that the wife of the person on our hospice said that whenever one of our team members would pull up in the driveway, Oscar would go to the door and wait. This included the first time our social worker dropped in for the initial consult. The woman said what was unusual was that when anyone else arrived, Oscar always barked, whether it was a family member or stranger. However, when I arrived for the first visit, having never been there before, Oscar went to the door and waited. The woman said, "I knew you were with hospice because he didn't bark." She said she had no idea how the little guy could discern who was with hospice and who wasn't.

The second interesting thing about Oscar was that when the wife would walk over to the couch, Oscar would jump on the arm, then spring up to the back of the couch and lie down as the wife would sit. He would act as a pillow for her. He only did this for her. I knew that I was accepted by Oscar when, after the fourth or fifth visit, as I went to sit on the couch, Oscar jumped on the arm of the couch and sprang up to the back and acted as a pillow for me.

Yes, dogs are affected by the passing of their owners. One evening one of our nurses, Mary, was called to a home because the final hour had come for a man on service. Mary entered the home moments after the man passed. Consoling the spouse, she noticed that the normally happy, active dog was curled up behind her owner's favorite recliner, whimpering. If dogs cry, this dog was crying. She was definitely grieving. This incident reminded me of how the caring staff of hospice is concerned with all who are affected by the illness and the passing. The fact that Mary brought this ostensibly insignificant incident to light emphasizes it.

I haven't mentioned cats too much, but they are also an important part of a family's life. My family has a house cat, Sammy, but his main concern focuses on where he's going to sleep. It may not be obvious, but Sammy and all cats are observant. They know when the routine of their household is changing. And believe it or not, cats also understand our nonverbal communication extremely well and may offer comfort in times of crisis.

Understanding there is a strong emotional connection between a family and their pets, most hospices will make sure pets are a part of the discussion when developing a plan of care. Pets are included.

Pets Can Be A Part of the Plan

ONE OF THE hallmarks of my hospice and many others is that we pay attention to everyone affected by the patient's condition. If desired, the entire family is included in the plan of care of the patient. And I mean everybody is included, even the pets.

As a patient-contact volunteer I accepted the assignment of a man who had a parakeet. While I would sit with the patient, the parakeet would talk to itself, saying "hello, hello," then occasionally saying a few different words. During one visit someone knocked on the door, and the parakeet started to make a noise sort of like a seal. I don't know how else to describe it.

I mentioned the noise to the man's wife when she came home. She started to laugh. She said the previous summer, she and her husband had gone on vacation and had taken the parakeet to stay at a family member's house. That family owned a dog that barked when someone knocked on the door. Evidently the parakeet learned to bark when someone knocked on the door. Like any good "bird dog," the parakeet was letting me know someone was at the door. I guess everyone wants to get into the act.

Several years ago I was making a marketing call to a large medical practice. Upon arrival I went back to the employees' lunchroom, where I was to make my presentation. A nurse was there, eating an early lunch. She saw my hospice name badge and immediately began to tell me about an experience that she had at the Pickering House, our in-patient facility.

She told me that her family was holding a vigil at her

grandma's bedside at the Pickering House, and by 4:00 a.m., all had dozed off. Our Pickering House cat, Chester, was in the room. Chester is also everyone's pet when they are at the Pickering House. He had been quiet and off to the side, but he began to meow. That caused the nurse to stir but not fully awaken. Suddenly Chester, who had been near her feet, pounced on her lap, startling her. The nurse noticed that the grandmother was barely breathing, so she woke up the family. The grandma died within a few minutes. Chester then quietly walked out.

One of the interesting things about this episode is that it happened over a year before I entered the employees' lunchroom. Yet, it was the first thought on the nurse's mind when she saw me. What Chester did really made an impression on her. All I could tell her is that Chester is there when needed.

Not to exclude the dogs, I had a patient who had a Schnauzer. The dog, Shultz, always needed to be let out at 7:00 p.m. I thought the patient's dad was being silly, but as he and his wife were preparing to leave for dinner, he would kneel down and tell Shultz, "Remember to tell Rick to let you out at 7:00 p.m." Schultz would bark once. Sure enough, a few minutes before 7:00 p.m., Shultz would bark once, then go to the back door. He always got his treat when he came back in. He was a nice diversion for the family, who were losing their son. Makes me wonder who trained who in this situation.

Pets do become a part of the family. They can offset sadness and give joy and, yes, create problems. Not only are they there to be a part of their family's end-of-life crisis, but they also teach about life and death. Pet owners know that someday their pets will die, most likely before they do. The pleasure of pets compensates for the pain of eventual loss. Through the pain of losing a pet, children learn death is a part of life. As painful as a pet's loss is, it helps us deal with more difficult losses ahead.

Hospice understands that pets enrich our lives. We let them be a part of our care plan because they will pitch in to do what they can when the family needs them the most.

Even Cats Sometimes Help

IN EVERY AREA of health care, the paramount focus of the medical staff is obviously the illness. When an appointment begins, the health-care professional may ask a few general questions about you or your family, but then it's down to business. With our health-care system, it is the way it has to be. There is only time for them to focus on the illness.

People consider hospice to be the last stage of the health-care continuum. The last house on the block, so to speak. I'm here to assure you we are not. We are not even on the same street. The last specialist you visited is actually your last stop on the health-care continuum, i.e., the last house on the block. Hospice's focus is completely different from a normal health-care professional's focus. We do not focus on the illness; we focus on the person who is ill. Asking about you and your family helps us to develop your plan of care. We'll even ask about your pets if you have any.

Many times pets will help us if we pay attention to them. In one particular instance, a man on my hospice had an indoor cat. As a person with a cat, I know that there are no ordinary cats. This cat soon proved he was a smart cat even though, like the typical unassuming cat, he never let on that he was interested in anything but sleeping.

The man's son told me of his last visit with his dad. He was being cared for in his home. He liked to be a part of the action and didn't want to be sequestered back in his bedroom. In order to be kept "in the loop," he had his bed placed where the couch had been in the living room.

On this particular evening, the family had gathered at the

house because the man's health was declining at a noticeable rate. He became tired, so family and friends, who had gathered, moved to the kitchen to allow him to quietly rest. About twenty minutes later, the conversation in the kitchen was suddenly interrupted by the family cat. It came running into the kitchen from the living room and, as one of the family members put it, "Just threw a fit. There's no other way to describe it; he just threw a fit."

At first, no one could figure out what was wrong with the cat, but someone suggested that they had better go into the living room to check on things. Very quickly they noticed the man's breathing pattern had changed. This was not a good indication. Months earlier, when the man had signed onto hospice care, his nurse had explained to the family the sequence in which certain things may happen as the body begins the normally slow process of turning itself off.

After the family went to the living room, they noticed the man had begun Cheyne-Stokes (pronounced "chain stokes") breathing, signaling the end was near.

The family called the hospice office to let them know what was going on, then pulled up chairs around the bed and sat in silent prayer. In less than an hour, the man died. Now they understood that the cat sensed the end was very close and was trying to get everyone's attention.

As I mentioned, hospice's focus is not on the illness, but on the patient. We include the family pet in the care plan since pets are a part of the family. Sometimes the pet may become a little more involved, as this cat was, and that is fine with us. We know that even cats sometimes help.

Dogs Just Know

Quite a few years ago as a hospice volunteer, I accepted the assignment of Harold, a man in his late 70's. He was on service due to kidney failure. He lived in a small cabin with his small dog, a pug. Arriving for my first visit, I knocked on the door. His dog started to bark and Harold told me to come in. The dog ran alongside of the couch to the other end of the room where the man was sitting in a recliner. He petted the dog which then lay at his feet.

The man told me that I must be "A good fellow" because his little dog didn't fuss when I came in. I told him the Volunteer Manager alerted me to the fact that his dog was blind so how would his little female pug know if I was good or bad? All the man said was that "Dogs just know".

Towards the end of my visit someone knocked on the door and his little dog got up and started to bark. Since she was blind I assumed that she only uses one way to go to the door and back. Well, she ran towards the door on the side of the room opposite the way she ran when I came in. Suddenly, "bam!" she ran headlong into my leg. She yelped and ran back to Harold. I felt bad because it startled the dog but the man thought it was funny saying, "Yes, my dog knows but she just doesn't know everything."

Then in a serious tone of voice he told me because of her he was able to live much longer than he should have. He said that several years ago his dog began sniffing around just above his waist line and would whine. He said that after a while he was getting annoyed by it and casually mentioned the dog's behavior to his doctor during a semi-annual checkup. His doctor was concerned because it is thought that dogs can sometimes smell certain diseases inside a human's body.

It turned out to be a kidney problem that, due to early detection, was able to be controlled for a few years. Harold told me that when he said dogs just know, he didn't know how the do but he is so thankful they do.

True Comfort

Years ago, we went to the rescue dog shelter to see what animals needed a home. My daughter saw a little brown and beige puppy in the back of the kennel, shivering in fright. "We'll take that one." With that, Rusty became one of our family. All his life he was absolutely petrified of other dogs. He was never able to get over the trauma of his time at the rescue shelter.

I was reminded of that recently when one of my hospice's social workers told me of a man on hospice who was brought to our inpatient facility, the Pickering House, to give his wife a break from his constant care. His family, as mine, had a pet that was a rescue dog. Even though the family knew pets were welcome to stay with family at the facility, they thought it best to keep her home. It seems that for whatever reason, the dog wouldn't go into unfamiliar buildings. The family thought the fear was because of something that had happened to her as a puppy.

The family quickly realized the little one needed her owner. She just kept whimpering. When they brought the dog out to see the man staying at the Pickering House, sure enough, she wouldn't go inside. So our staff wheeled the bedridden man outside and the little dog lit up, jumping up on the bed and excitedly licking her owner's face in a nonstop frenzy.

Hospice is well known for comforting the people under their care. But anyone with a dog will tell you that nothing can replace the simple act of your dog licking your face and the joy of being reunited with your pet. That is true comfort.

A Metal Folding Chair

There is nothing new under the sun, even in today's world. For example, take isolating people when they are suffering from or are vulnerable to certain illnesses. Going back to biblical times, people afflicted with leprosy were isolated from contact with the general population. With the advancement of technology, we now have many options to choose from when contacting someone who is isolated due to fear of infection, three prevalent avenues being phone, Skype, or Zoom. These are, however, stopgap measures, and they ignore our need for physical human contact.

During the twenty-plus years of my association with hospice, I have heard of several occasions where we were restricted in our contact with the person on service, either due to the symptoms of the person's illness or those of a family member. A while ago, I was conversing with one of our volunteers, Pat. He told me of one of his most unusual experiences as a patient-contact volunteer. Yes, it involved being isolated from the person on service, but he certainly wasn't excluded.

Before he accepted the assignment of the man (always the volunteer's option), Pat learned the person on service and his wife, both in their eighties, were still living in their house. The couple was blessed to have a large, loving family, all of whom helped whenever needed. As the couple's health started to decline, the family devised a plan that would allow the couple to continue living in their home. Each sibling would stay with the parents for a twenty-four-hour shift. That worked out to be one day a week for each of the kids, the kids themselves being in their fifties and sixties. This arrangement allowed each child to assist his or her parents for only one day a week, allowing the other siblings to carry on their lives as normally as they could. It worked well.

Eventually the husband became terminally ill. His wife, with her developing frailties, was not able to care for her husband anymore. Ironically, at first glance, the husband seemed to be the healthier of the two.

Hospice was called. Soon the house was a hive of activity as the family gathered and prepared for the changes that were taking place. One change occurred when the dad asked if he could have his bed placed in the center of the front window. He said he "still wanted to be a part of the action." As the couple wanted to remain close to one another, the wife's bed was positioned next to his. Her bed was to the right of the window and out of sight.

Once the husband was settled, our social worker mentioned a volunteer was available to stop by to visit if desired. Hearing about that option, the family strongly suggested to their dad that he should take advantage of the offer. Evidently their dad was a storyteller, and his family said they had all heard his stories more than once. However, the man's wife had pulmonary problems, which precluded anyone from visiting without a complete head-to-toe personal protective suit. The family said they "didn't want an astronaut to visit." So, they would try to find a solution. They did, and a volunteer visit was arranged.

On his first visit, our volunteer, Pat, noticed a standard metal folding chair on the sidewalk connecting the driveway to the front porch. The man's daughter met Pat at the door. She asked if he would mind sitting on the chair placed about ten feet from the window and use his cell phone to call her dad. That way her dad could see Pat as they talked, and her mom would be safe from any contact from people outside. It was a simple idea, and many conversations were had from that point forward.

The two turned out to be a perfect match. Pat said the conversations were probably the most interesting he's ever had with someone on service and definitely in the most interesting setting. To the casual observer, seeing a man sitting on a small metal folding chair, looking at a house while talking on the phone, was definitely one of those "What the . . . ." moments.

The only requirement for hospice care is a prognosis of six months or less of life. And most hospices will help no matter what your circumstances. However, would you mind keeping a metal folding chair handy just in case?

Not Around When Not Needed

Probably what impresses families the most when they first accept hospice care is the completely focused interest in the person and their family given by the hospice staff. Being so focused helps hospice staff to learn the likes and dislikes of the person on service enabling them to develop a plan of care around them. After all, it is their life and at this stage freedom of choice is very important.

In the early years of my volunteering, I accepted the assignment of a man in his late 70's named "Hank". During the late 1940s he had been a car salesman. As luck would have it, I have a collection of magazine car ads from that time period. I keep the car ads in several large scrap books.

On one particular afternoon, Hank was scheduled to have a visit from his hospice nurse. The purpose was to stop by for a simple checkup. At the last minute he declined the visit. I had called him that morning and asked him would he mind if I stopped over with my scrap books containing the car ads. He excitedly said he'd love it.

The nurse later explained that she knew the family well enough that if either Hank or his daughter felt a visit was necessary she would have stopped by.

Hank commented to me as we were thumbing through the old car ad pages that, "What I like about you people is that you don't hang around here when I don't need ya."

After completing this story, I didn't think I should title it, "Hang Around Here When I Don't Need Ya". So, "Not Around When Not Needed" will have to do.

Do Something with That Hair

When I was training to become a hospice volunteer, an area of opportunity that I never dreamed would be a part of hospice volunteering was giving haircuts. After all, the assumption tends to be if you sign onto hospice, the end is right around the corner. So why would anyone need a haircut? It seems like such a little thing to be concerned about when big things are happening. Yet in life it is often the little things we remember years later, rather than the big things.

Understandably, if someone has been fighting a disease for an extended amount of time, the person's hair most likely has been neglected or has probably not even been thought of. That makes sense because when someone is extremely ill, everyone's focus is on eliminating the disease and restoring health. This is precisely what differentiates hospice care from curative care. Hospice doesn't focus on the disease. Our focus is on the person.

By placing the center of our attention on the person's hair, it redirects the focus, if only for a little bit, from the disease. This focus signifies the one who is ill is still thinking externally, and his or her appearance matters to the person. Attention to a person's hair implies the individual is still here, and the person still wants to look good.

Gwen, a licensed hairstylist, is one of our volunteers who has for many years been giving those on our hospice either a fresh haircut or styling their hair. She said, especially for those people experiencing hospice, one of the reasons to give time and attention to someone's hair is how it makes the recipient feel, to a degree, that life is returning to normal. People are able to enjoy a routine that has been a part of their entire life.

The whole atmosphere changes in a room when someone is having his or her hair done. The stories of first haircuts, eighties hairstyles, and, of course, high school yearbook pictures, bring lively discussions and laughter. Gwen told me it never seems to fail that while she is cutting or styling hair, she will always hear someone comment about how the recipient will be charming the opposite sex.

During the last stage of life, the little things become the big things. Although our volunteer brochure may not mention it, someone may have the opportunity to volunteer in ways he or she never expected. Even if it is to "do something with that hair."

Fairly early in my time as a patient-contact volunteer I accepted the assignment of a man, "Jimmy," who was in his early forties. He was afflicted with AIDS and had been revoked, or not accepted, by several hospices in the Central Ohio area. It was during the late 1990s, and the fear of contracting AIDS was still prevalent.

As I got to know Jimmy, I began to understand why he was having so much trouble with other hospice agencies agreeing to provide his care; he definitely had a chip on his shoulder. The hospice I am associated with adapts to the wants and needs of each of those on service, and Jimmy was one who required a lot of adapting on our part. He was accepted by our staff and placed under our care.

Jimmy was on our hospice for quite a while, and over time he, too, needed to do something with his hair. He asked me if I could give him a haircut. I jokingly told him that if I gave him one, he'd need to wear a hat. My initial thought, like most people, was that haircuts aren't in our realm, but I told him I would ask my volunteer coordinator what our options were. The coordinator said she knew of no one at that time with barbering experience but suggested I look around for one.

I called several retired barbers I knew and asked if they would cut the hair of a bedridden hospice patient. Each one said they had no problem doing that, even though the person on hospice lived in a county not in our normal service area. They were willing, that is until I mentioned that Jimmy had AIDS. Then, one by one, each gave, in sometimes lengthy dissertations, reasons why they couldn't, saying they "lost their clippers" or "I'll have to ask my wife." Excuse after excuse was given.

In desperation, I called my church's office. The church has a large congregation, so I thought there would be a barber, retired or active, who would be willing to cut Jimmy's hair. When I called Suanne at the parish office, she said she was sure we had someone who could do it, but offhand, no one immediately came to mind. Then she asked if there was anything she could do to help as she had experience with cutting hair. She said she was the only one who cut her children's hair, noting, "They all lived through it!"

I explained I had accepted a volunteer assignment for a man who needed a haircut. Suanne immediately said that she could help. I explained that he lived in the next county, a full half-hour's drive away. She said it was no problem; she could do it. Then I dropped "the bomb." I told her Jimmy had AIDS. Suanne merely asked what his address was. I started to repeat myself to make sure she fully understood what she was agreeing to, and Suanne interrupted me, saying emphatically, "If he needs help, I'll help. It's just that simple."

Not only did she cut Jimmy's hair, but she stayed for an extra half hour just to talk with him. In addition, she stayed to talk to his parents. No one, siblings, friends, or retired barbers, had wanted to help this man until Suanne. Jimmy's dad said what he witnessed reminded him of Matthew 25:40, "Amen, I say to you, whatever you did for one of these least brothers of Mine, you did for Me."

Years later I was talking to Jimmy's parents about their experience with hospice. Both mentioned how the attention given to him at the end of his life from strangers lifted and carried his parents through the years long after his passing. His dad said when hospice came in, their son was accepted, pure and simple. His mom said she couldn't imagine "that woman" drove so far just to cut Jimmy's hair, adding, "She was so nice." So many years later, the haircut is what stood out. In life, it is always the small things that are remembered.

Graduations

Late spring is the season for the majority of graduations, and graduations are a part of life. Who knows more about the seasons of life than an organization that assists people at the end of theirs? And since I am talking about graduations, maybe I should mention that, yes, we in the hospice field have a lot of experience with graduations. Say what? Hospice graduates patients? Yes, when someone's health improves to the point where a person no longer meets the Medicare requirement of a six-month-or-less prognosis, then we revoke, or graduate, individuals from our care.

In essence, such people are just too healthy to be on hospice service. That, in the business, is known as "graduating" from hospice. I've always said that if I'm going to graduate from anything, I want to graduate from hospice.

Thinking of some of those whom my hospice has graduated, one woman who immediately comes to mind lived in an area nursing home. Her name was Gladys, and she was one hundred and two years old. Before she came onto hospice, Gladys was, in her own words, "beginning to wear out." Well, as statistics from the past forty years have consistently shown, when a person is on hospice service early enough in what is considered the last stage of life, the individual's health tends to improve. And whether a person's health improves or just stabilizes, all studies have shown people live longer while on hospice than their doctors had originally thought, the exception being those who are referred to us with only hours of life remaining.

Since Gladys was thrilled to be graduating from hospice, her nurse, Tammy, thought it would be nice to have a full-fledged graduation ceremony. With our social worker coordinating with the nursing home staff, the ceremony was planned. The residents of the nursing home were excited and couldn't wait for the great celebration.

One of the nursing home dining rooms was decorated in a graduation theme by Gladys's children, grandchildren, great-grandchildren, and even a few great-great-grandchildren. A special cake was prepared by kitchen staff, and invitations were sent. For her big day, Gladys wore a cap and gown and was brought into the dining room while a recording of "Pomp and Circumstance" played. Nursing home staff, hospice staff, and her family all cheered. Gladys was elated.

She received a certificate of graduation from the CEO, Denise Bauer, who said, "I wouldn't miss this event for the world. It is so wonderful to see such a large turnout of family and friends. And look at all of these great-grandchildren. This is what hospice is all about."

In a very unique way, another person on our hospice was involved in, I guess you'd say, a "graduation situation," but with a pleasantly unexpected result. She was in her late seventies. The social worker who was admitting her onto hospice asked her, as our social workers ask each new admission, if she had any hopes, dreams, regrets, etc. Yes, in fact, the woman did have a regret. She said that during World War II she had dropped out of high school in her senior year so she could work in one of the war factories.

After the war, the woman felt she was too old to go back to high school. She eventually earned her GED certificate. She got married and raised her family. Now, all these years later, she was signing onto hospice and entering into what looked like her last few months of life. She still regretted not receiving her high school diploma. So often the significance of an event is not known until it becomes a memory.

The regret this woman felt about not obtaining her high school diploma bothered the social worker. Soon he got the idea to write the woman's old high school, which was several states away, to find out if they would consider awarding her a diploma, possibly an honorary one. After all, she had dropped out of school for patriotic reasons and had completed her school work by earning her GED.

The high school thought it was a great idea and agreed. Soon, the woman had her diploma in hand. She was so proud. She showed her children, grandchildren, and great-grandchildren. Everyone was happy for her, including the hospice staff. And as they say in the TV infomercials, "But wait, there's more!"

Several weeks later, the woman received a letter from her high school's alumni association. It was an invitation to her sixtieth high school reunion. She was included! Since she never graduated from high school, she had never registered as an alumnus and, therefore, had never received a class reunion invitation. The woman had long ago given up on the idea of attending her class reunion, even though she had been with her classmates through over eleven years of school. Besides, she had moved far away and lost track of everyone.

What a wonderful feeling it was for her to be included after sixty years! That was the real reward. The simple gesture of being invited to her class reunion made her feel like she had truly graduated with her classmates.

When hospice says that we celebrate life, it demonstrates that philosophy through efforts to help its patients celebrate the milestones of their life. We assist those on our hospice to eliminate any regrets and enjoy the last stage of life. Every hospice knows that nothing is really over until you stop trying. Life is not over until a person gives up on living. We encourage and, most importantly, assist those under our care in truly living and celebrating their lives. We don't think spending the last stage of life trying not to die is a good idea.

When graduating from any school, college, or yes, even hospice, realize this, too, is a commencement. You are commencing a new stage in your life. I hope you understand, appreciate, and live life. It's been said many times that we should enjoy the little things because at some point we will look back and realize they were the big things.

She Left as She Came

We enter this world with no concerns or earthly possessions. I've heard many times that one of the pathways to peace and serenity is to go full circle and let go of all concerns and earthly possessions at some point in your life. Not long ago, my hospice signed a pragmatic woman onto our service who very poignantly confirmed those two statements. Her illness was incurable, and instead of fighting it to the bitter end (and have people proud of her for doing so), she decided to sign onto hospice and enjoy as much as possible her last stage of life.

Once settled into her new routine of living and not going anywhere for another treatment, the woman decided to give her valuables to her adult children. She was allowed the gift of seeing their reaction as they received their inheritance. She also received a lot of enjoyment watching her children be given the possessions that held so many memories. There were a lot of stories and much laughter as the possessions were passed down to her children. After the woman gave away those items, she arranged for an auction company to sell her remaining items. She was now completely free of any earthly possessions and ready to meet her Creator.

The only problem was that her Creator was not quite ready to meet her. As often happens when someone signs onto hospice soon after being told of their six-month prognosis, the woman's health improved. No longer appropriate for hospice, she signed off of service. She moved in with her son and, as I heard later, lived a very happy, carefree life. And, I might add, with no earthly concerns or possessions.

Time passed, and the woman eventually signed back on to our service. With her children at her bedside, she died in her sleep the next day. This woman truly left this life the same way that she entered, with nothing and not a care in the world.

Celebrating the Lasts

MANY HOSPICES WILL say, "We celebrate life." That is not just a catchy phrase. During this stage of life, those involved in hospice care help those on our service honor and celebrate their life. One of the ways we help people to celebrate life is to recognize the lasts they have experienced in their life, and we help them to celebrate those occurrences.

One of our volunteers once mentioned one of the honors of being a patient-contact volunteer is the fact that most likely he will be the last "new" person that the individual on our service will ever meet or be introduced to. I had not thought about that, but it is probably true.

This got me thinking about how many people I have met in my life and how many more I have yet to meet. And by meeting people, I mean either being formally introduced or interacting with them in some capacity. How many people does an ordinary person meet during his or her entire life? Fifteen thousand? Thirty thousand? Studies have estimated that we may have contact with as many as one hundred and twenty thousand different people during a lifetime.

It has been said that time decides who you meet in life, your heart decides who you want in your life, and your behavior decides who stays in your life. So, I guess a variation of that question would be to ask, "How many people will you impact during your life?" I know that I have made some people happy by entering a room and others by leaving a room.

When you think about it, starting at birth, you were (sort of) introduced to your mother and father, then to your immediate family, then to aunts and uncles, cousins, and gradually to friends, teachers, clergy, coaches, spouse(s), in-laws, coworkers, neighbors, and medical personnel. Finally, should you choose hospice, you meet your care team.

The volunteer is usually the last person on the hospice team the person may meet. The volunteer I mentioned above said he tries to treat everyone he is introduced to as the last person he will ever meet. He said as a volunteer he is honored to be that person. That seems to emphasize the importance of "lasts" as much as "firsts."

Our society celebrates the firsts in life, but it usually doesn't celebrate the lasts because we don't know when they will occur. We celebrate a baby's first word, but what about the last word uttered before the dying process finishes its course? We celebrate a baby's first step, but when was the last step taken as an adult, before he couldn't get out of bed anymore? We celebrate the first time a baby puts the spoon in her mouth all by herself, but when was the last time she fed herself before illness left her too weak to lift the spoon?

Personally, I remember the thrill I experienced the first time as a little boy learning to ride a bike, when I broke away from my dad, who was running alongside me, and rode a two-wheeler by myself. But when did I park my bicycle in the garage as a teenager for the last time? That also was a milestone and one of those subtle transitions from childhood to adulthood. And when was the last time I played hide-and-seek with my friends in the neighborhood? Although I must admit, I do remember leaving high school on the last day as a senior and celebrating that "last" life event.

My first job was at the Fairborn Theatre in Fairborn, Ohio. After all of the times I went there as a kid to watch a movie, it was strange to think that I would be working there. I'll never forget opening the door of the theater when beginning my first day on the job, the first day of my working career.

I'm guessing being part of hospice will be my last job. There has been a lot of punching my time card between my first job and now. (I'll explain what "punching my time card" means to the younger folks another time.)

The hospice medical staff understand how the body slowly turns itself off during the last stage of life. As the process begins, our staff will explain to the family when each of the subtle changes has happened. Months later someone from the family will tell us how important it was to know when a last-time event happened and how profound it was.

Not too long ago, one of the lasts that a man on service and his family got to experience was their last Thanksgiving dinner. With the assistance of FAIRHOPE staff and volunteers, it was held at the Pickering House. The person on service said how much he had always loved Thanksgiving dinner, especially his son-in-law's homemade noodles.

Well, even though it was summertime, we encouraged the family to have a "last supper," so to speak, and celebrate. The family brought in all the ingredients and fixed Thanksgiving dinner in the Pickering House's family kitchen. Our staff set up a long banquet table in the family dining room. The patient and family had a wonderful Thanksgiving dinner in August.

In another instance, a husband and wife, with the help of FAIRHOPE Hospice staff and volunteers, were able to celebrate their fifty-eighth wedding anniversary at home, surrounded by their family, just hours before the husband died.

In a third example, we were able to help a son and his dad go fishing together one last time before the dad died.

Pain and discomfort are a part of being ill. This may become your entire focus to the point that you may lose sight of the life you still have ahead of you. You will not realize a "for the last time" event has passed. Hospice allows the families of those on service to celebrate the lasts.

Commemorating the lasts is not as much about dwelling on the past as it is about honoring it. At the same time, there is still life ahead. Celebrate it before it's too late.

A Freeing Experience

ONE OF THE prevalent misconceptions about hospice is that the patient is going to die soon if he or she signs on. But sometimes people don't. Their health may improve, and although they may still be terminally ill, they are no longer appropriate for hospice. If that is the case, hospice "graduates" such individuals from service.

A while ago my hospice signed a pragmatic woman onto service. Instead of fighting her incurable illness to the bitter end and having people be proud of her for doing so, she decided to stop treatments and enjoy the last stage of her life as much as her disease would allow. The hospice team helped her develop a care plan to manage her illness. As sometimes happens when someone accepts hospice care soon enough, the woman's health actually improved, and she was well enough to be graduated from hospice care.

She settled into a new routine of living life to its fullest. No more traveling for appointments and treatments. The woman was in charge and decided now was the right time to give her valuables to her children, thus allowing her to see their reaction rather than leaving the items in her will. Then she made plans for an auction company to sell her remaining possessions, and she sold her home. The woman was now free of any earthly possessions and ready to meet her Creator. The only problem was that her Creator was not ready to meet her.

Who knows if selling everything she owned released her from the burden of material concerns, or if the all-encompassing hospice care contributed to her longer-than-expected life. The fact was that by accepting her illness, not allowing it to control her life, and by making her own choices, the woman's last stage of life was happy, joyous, and free.

It is Spiritual

WHEN SOMEONE ACCEPTS hospice service, a unique plan of care is developed by inquiring about the person's physical, emotional, and spiritual needs. Up until the point of calling hospice, the focus has been almost exclusively on a person's physical symptoms and emotional health. The end of life, however, has its own nature and now warrants a complete reorganization of priorities.

As the last stage of life progresses, the initial concern is pain control and then addressing any emotional distress. Lastly, the person's spiritual needs become paramount.

For each new person on service, one of our chaplains will always make a phone call to inquire if there are any spiritual needs or questions. A visit is offered. I don't know what our chaplains' overall batting average is, but sometimes the person wants a visit, and sometimes he or she doesn't. Should someone decline the offer, the chaplain doesn't give a "sales pitch." It is the person's life and his or her choice. We respect that.

Talking to one of our chaplains, he said that when it comes to a spiritual belief system in our southeast Ohio area, Christianity is the predominant spiritual belief system. He surprised me, however, by saying when inquiring about a person's spiritual beliefs, he has encountered a total of 16 different belief systems. These include the Jewish tradition and two different Native American belief traditions.

If requested, hospice chaplains will assist a person's clergy or spiritual leader in giving the person the spiritual comfort he or she needs. Sometimes, however, it seems the spirits themselves step in to administer comfort. The first such "spiritual encounter" at our in-patient facility occurred, ironically, when a woman, "Virginia," who graciously donated enough financial assistance to allow construction to begin on our in-patient facility, was spending her remaining days there.

In late morning, our housekeeper, Pat D., was at work in Virginia's room. Pat noticed her seemingly looking through the ceiling. Virginia said, "I can't come yet, Daddy." She then looked at Pat, saying, "Daddy said he wants me to come up."

Within 24 hours, Virginia was up with her daddy.

As I was completing this book, a spiritual event occurred in the same facility. Our hospice house charge nurse, Heidi, told me that an hour ago, the man in Room 8 had sat up in bed and casually started talking to his daughter. Since he had been in a deep sleep for several days, his sudden awakening startled his daughter. She was his only visitor at the time. He told her that he needed to get ready for a journey.

"Where to?" his daughter asked.

"You can't go. When you leave, I am going to go on a journey," he replied. He said he was going to go on a journey so he could be with "Jeanette," his wife who had died years before. After a while, he asked his daughter if she could "see them" as he gazed out his room's window.

"See who?" his daughter asked.

"All those angels out there. Open the window so they can come in." She did.

The daughter then said her father started to talk to "Miles," who was near the room's door. She said no one was in the corner. She asked who Miles was, and I don't think her father answered her, but he kept talking to Miles. The daughter said no one in the family knew of a Miles. A little research in Hebrew Baby Names revealed the name Miles's meaning is "Who is like God? Gift from God."

When anyone discusses spirituality with someone at the end of life, it seems to be more of a question-and-answer type of conversation. And the topics are based more on what we've been taught. Every so often it is the person preparing to cross over who leads the discussion. And when the person leads the discussion, it *is* spiritual.

CHAPTER 3
The Ache Begins

"One of the most important things you can do on this Earth is to let people know they are not alone."

—Shannon L. Alder

This Gift is from My Sister

Setting up a display is one of many outreach activities hospice utilizes to allow both professionals and the general public to meet staff and get a better understanding of what we do. A considerable amount of thought goes into planning our display. For my hospice, the many compliments about our display confirm that we put our best into everything we do, even the ostensibly little things.

We set up at large conferences, county fairs, and everywhere in between. And yes, by being at public events, people who have experienced our compassion will come up and thank us. Personally, I love working at our display table because I learn the importance and the effectiveness of hospice during a time of unthinkable crisis.

One event we recently attended as a vendor was a conference held in Columbus, Ohio. This particular event happened to be a statewide conference for the health-care community. It involved a series of educational presentations with breaks between each session. During these breaks, the attendees would visit the displays of various organizations. My hospice was one of several hospices present. Beth, our education manager, and Kim, our community educator, were our representatives at this conference. It was a well-attended event, and the two were kept busy as quite a few people stopped to talk.

During this event, one participant stood out. Initially, she was very hesitant to approach our display table. She stood across the aisle and gazed at the display, not making eye contact with either Kim or Beth. My personal experience at these events has taught me that those who don't understand hospice usually want to keep it that way. They normally approach our display, take one of our giveaway pens and a Post-it note, and keep moving. Rarely does anyone without hospice experience make eye contact with us.

In this case, Kim's intuition told her this woman needed to talk. Obviously, just giving her one of our snazzy giveaway pens was out of the question. Moving around to the front of our table, Kim introduced herself. She quickly learned the woman's name was "Teresa." Through reddening eyes, she said her sister had died on our hospice about six months ago.

Teresa said she still talked to her sister every day and knew she was watching over her. Kim nodded in agreement. Teresa said she had hoped the intensity of the grief she was feeling would lessen. Instead, it seemed to have steadily gotten worse. Staring at our display brought back a series of intense memories. Picking up anything with the word "hospice" on it was impossible for her. Beth assured her we were always available if she needed to talk.

After their conversation, in which Kim and Beth did most of the listening, Teresa hesitantly put her business card in our large glass bowl for the door prize drawing. After a deep sigh, she walked away. That was it; a conversation that lasted only moments.

Yes, Kim and Beth were at the conference to educate. But foremost, the purpose of all hospice staff is to comfort. Setting up a display gives us the opportunity to do just that. It doesn't matter if we set up a display at a 5K fundraiser, a county fair, or a statewide health-care conference; our primary purpose is always to offer comfort. At the very least, while at our display, Teresa was able to talk to two people who sympathetically listened.

As the conference was coming to a close, each vendor dutifully brought up a container of business cards for the door prize drawings. Our door prize consisted of an oversized gift basket filled with comfort items such as bath salts, lavender bath oils, wine, waffle slippers, body lotions, bubble bath, and quite a few more similar items. To Beth, it looked as if every attendee put a card in the bowl. She estimated over two hundred business cards were in our container. "Obviously, we were offering a popular door prize," she told me.

With a lot of fanfare, the emcee reached into the box containing the names of each of the many vendors who had donated a door prize. As it happened, we were the first vendor chosen to select a door prize drawing. Next, a randomly chosen attendee reached into our glass bowl, took out a business card, and gave it to Beth to announce the winner.

Beth stared at the card as if she was having a hard time reading it. This was one of those times in life when there are no words. There, on the business card, was Teresa's name! Kim felt a shiver when she heard Teresa's name called. Beth and Kim looked at each other. There just couldn't have been a more perfect prize for a more deserving person! They will tell you that there was no doubt that a spiritual event just occurred.

A backstory to this day is that, months ago, there had been quite a long discussion as to the need for attending this conference. This was a statewide event, and the majority of attendees would be located outside of our coverage area, with some coming from several hundred miles away. We went anyway, setting up our display at an event where a shrewd business person would say we had little potential for viable contacts. Our purpose is to be available to comfort all who need it. At this event, someone who needed consoling was consoled. By our standards, the event was a success.

And to think that just a few short hours prior, Teresa didn't want to put her card in the container for the drawing. She didn't want anything from us or any hospice. In an ironic turn of events, when presented with the basket, Teresa said it was the best gift she ever could have received.

Yes, death ends a life, but it doesn't end a relationship. Love never dies. Between tears, Teresa told Beth and Kim, "This gift is from my sister." Evidently, Teresa's sister needed to borrow Beth and Kim. She needed for them to be the facilitators to let Teresa know her sister was still with her, watching over her as sisters always do.

Where She Needed to Be

I was at the memorial service of a mother who had been on our hospice. I was talking to her daughter, who told me her mother had requested to be cremated when she died, so no traditional funeral was held. Standing there at the service reminded me of a saying in the funeral industry, "A good funeral gets the dead where they need to go and the living where they need to be."

One of the benefits of calling hours or visitation at a traditional funeral is that the family and friends get to see the deceased one last time. And if I can be gentle about it, the deceased look more presentable at a funeral home than they do immediately after they die. The funeral tends to finalize that the person's body is dead, not just that they've "gone" somewhere. This is very important for children.

Part of what hospice does, whether plans are made for a traditional funeral or not, is to get the living where they need to be from an emotional point of view. We accomplish this by taking the time to learn what the ill person and his or her family really care about and listening to what is important to them.

When the woman's mother died, the hospice nurse and the daughter were at her bedside. Knowing this would be the last time the daughter would get to see her mom, the hospice nurse, Heidi, quickly got to work. Heidi asked several nurse assistants to help her bathe and dress the mom's body in nice clothes. They put clean linens on the bed, combed the woman's hair, and put makeup on her. She looked natural and at rest.

It meant so much to the woman to witness the attention and respect given to her mom even after the woman had died. Heidi also indirectly showed respect to the daughter. In doing so, it created a good feeling and, given the circumstances, a wonderful memory. Truthfully, Heidi helped the daughter arrive at just where she needed to be.

A Thank-You Card

When someone sends a thank-you card to the hospice where I work, our medical team is given a chance to read it. I find it very refreshing to read those thank-you cards because it affirms that what we do in the hospice field has a positive effect on people during their time of unthinkable crisis.

One card in particular came from a woman whose mom spent a few days in the Pickering House (a free-standing hospice facility) for symptom management. She stated how her family felt more like guests in someone's home than like they were in any sort of medical facility. To be sure, our staff in the Pickering House view patients' families as our guests, not visitors.

Most of the thank-you cards don't specifically mention what impressed them because very few things that our staff does are profound; they are seemingly insignificant, thoughtful gestures that just accumulate. One card, however, did mention that one of our STNAs had done the woman's mom's nails "... in Mom's favorite color" only days before her passing. This simple gesture was the only specific thing mentioned in the thank-you card. Yes, she complimented us on our attentiveness and compassion. However, her mom's nails being tended to was the only act that was specifically mentioned; that was what the daughter noticed.

Every hospice staff member appreciates the gratitude people express, especially in a thank-you card. The card sublimely indicates a deeper gratitude because it must be purchased, a note written, and then mailed. That requires much more effort than a one-minute text.

Thank-you cards mean a lot to us because you and your family mean a lot to us.

Daylight Saving Time in Heaven

I'VE READ LOVE is a house that even death can't knock down. Well, at my hospice's most recent memorial service, I learned love may also help keep the house in order after death. I was talking to a man whose wife had been on our service. He told me not too long after his wife passed, he decided to put the house back in order. The medical equipment had been removed, and the sympathetic phone calls and visits had stopped, so now seemed to be the time.

Physically, it wasn't easy to do. Emotionally, it felt almost impossible. But eventually it was done. The night after the man had the house back in order, he awoke in the middle of the night with a jolt. His dog came running in to see what had happened. Nothing seemed unusual. Looking around, he noticed his alarm clock read 3:55 a.m.

The next morning, the man remembered that yesterday was the day in March when the clocks had been moved ahead one hour, meaning that technically, he was jolted awake at 4:55 a.m. Daylight Saving Time. He stared at the clock as he remembered his wife had died at 4:55 a.m. Realizing that, he smiled. Yes, she was reminding him to move the clock forward.

Even in his grief, the man felt assured his wife was telling him she was still in his life and, though gone physically, she would keep things in order. When she died, he didn't stop loving her, and she didn't stop loving him. Makes me wonder if they have Daylight Saving Time in heaven.

How Do You Do This?

Anyone who works or who has worked in the hospice field has heard the question, "How do you do this?" possibly followed by, "That is so morbid" or "That is so sad." Actually, working in hospice is a calling. It is one of those "Ya gotta wanna" endeavors. For those involved in end-of-life care, hospice is very meaningful and fulfilling.

One of our grief counselors, Ernie, is a retired pastor. He has heard all of the questions regarding why anyone would be involved with hospice. We had a fairly lengthy conversation where he told me why and how he can do this.

He said that in his more than thirty years of pastoring, he had never had someone ask him the question, "How can you do what you do?" i.e., be a pastor. Within three days of working in hospice, Ernie said, "I was asked a dozen times, 'How can you do what you do?'"

"I have pondered that question many times and feel like I have developed an answer that is consistent for both those grieving and for myself," he said. "My first response to the question is simply, 'I believe this is what God wants me to do.' My second response often catches people off guard; for a short time, we get to be God's hands extended to help families through one of the most difficult times of their lives."

Individuals are not alone when being served by hospice. He shared, "Now they have families and friends who are walking with them and feeling the same type of emotional pain they are experiencing. In working with a grieving family, I am able to normalize their feelings and emotions by giving them the freedom to express those emotions and feelings without judging them."

Not long ago, Ernie had a family member who expressed

they felt as if they were going crazy because they couldn't concentrate, stay focused, and was forgetting little things. Ernie told me these are all very normal during the grieving process. He had been meeting with the family on a regular basis. He said that after a time he was able to help alleviate most of the person's anxiousness and help them continue living. Ernie revealed, "To know that I was able to help someone in the depths of grieving is a joy, a satisfaction that can't be described."

At the end of our conversation, Ernie offered, "The real question shouldn't be why do I do this. It should be 'Why *wouldn't* I want to do this?'"

And Then Some

Hospice is not about medicine; it is about you. Without hospice support when someone enters the last stage of life, all focus is centered on the illness. Very little effort is dedicated to the wants and needs of the person who is ill or to the family's emotional needs. And there is little, or no thought given to what happens after the patient dies. "Not my problem" seems to be the extent of how most agencies address grief support after the passing. Part of that seemingly callous attitude is because grief counseling is not covered or is only minimally offered by insurance plans, nor is it a requirement for it to be included as a paid service for families by any government program.

Hospice's purpose is to deal with the physical, emotional, and spiritual needs of the patient and family before the passing and to maintain that effort with the family for over a year after the passing. It seems like when you leave the cemetery, it's all over. Everyone goes home. The phone calls offering to help have ceased, and you are encouraged to focus on adjusting to your new life. But think about it: just because a person's heart stops beating doesn't mean your heart stops loving.

The hospice grief support team understands that after the numbness and shock wear off, after all the "If there's anything I can do, just call me" statements have stopped, the real grief begins to develop. At this stage, the grieving family members are many times avoided because it is uncomfortable to be near them when they are grieving. It's at this time that hospice remains in contact with grieving family members with calls, letters, and visits for over a year after the passing.

And the best part is that some hospices, including where I work, don't charge for any of these essential, comforting grief support services. So, when your family enters into life's biggest crisis, know that hospice will assist you from beginning to end and then some.

Come Be With Me

How many heartfelt conversations have been shared sitting around a kitchen table? I'd like to share a moment one of our grief specialists experienced recently while having a nice conversation around the kitchen table with someone on our service and his spouse.

Tracey, one of our grief support coordinators, later sent me a note recapping the words of wisdom learned from this couple. Her story reads as follows:

> As we talked, I learned how phone calls and emails provided words of comfort and hope during the early days of learning to live with a life-limiting medical condition. I came to understand the importance of friends and family members continuing to be present and sharing hugs, laughter, tears, smiles, and silence throughout the ups and downs of a patient's journey.
>
> Unfortunately, many choose to stay away because they are uncertain what to say or are fearful of saying something wrong. As a result, family relationships and friendships suffer during a period of time when they are needed most.
>
> After talking to (the man) and his wife, I've learned what is most needed. They need to talk with you about times shared. They need to express joys and regrets. They need to be with you, sharing fears. They need to know that their life matters. They need to spend time alone with just you. They need to know and experience assurance that you will be present for their loved ones when they cannot.

Sharing this intimate time is a gift for all who choose to be present, unwrapping moment after moment. Call, visit, and give your time as a gift. In doing so, may you come to experience the joy that sharing such a gift can offer. It is never too late.

So, simply don't wait. Come be with me. It may just be what you both need.

CHAPTER 4
A Culture of Kindness

"If someone needs help, I help them.
It's that simple."

—Suanne G.

A Dad of Few Words

Hospice is a family-centered philosophy of care, meaning when we care for someone on service, we include the whole family. As a patient-contact volunteer, I am almost always matched with male patients. As I get to know men and their families, I always hear "dad stories." And dad stories seem to always involve the crazy things a man did and the lessons his family learned from him.

When it comes to men and dads in particular, they don't need to say much to communicate. Especially for dads, communicating is more a matter of simply being there. It is often quantity time over quality time. Growing up, I just liked Dad being home. I felt better when he was there. Dads tend to connect to us through their presence and by the things they do for our families.

One of the truths in life is that values are caught, not taught. This seems to be especially true with dads. I learned more from my dad by watching what he did than through any lectures. With him, results were not as important as effort. He was not a handyman, but he did try. That was a lesson caught: at least try. I still live by that mantra, and it is one of the many reasons that I find myself thinking that I am "just like Dad."

On weekends when Dad was home, I'd ask him if I could go with the neighborhood kids somewhere, such as to the woods. Dad would give me the okay, adding, "If you come back crying, you better be bleeding." I knew that reply gave me the freedom to just have fun and make my own decisions as to what to do, including doing something stupid once in a while. But I also knew if someone called me a name, not to worry about it. My dad was always teaching and guiding, but nurturing was Mom's department.

My dad demonstrated to me at an early age that if he asked me to do something, it was rarely a suggestion, nor was it a topic open for discussion. If I was told to do something, I should do it. Yet, he also instructed me that if someone asked me to do something I knew was wrong, I could confide in him.

The stature of a dad in the community isn't important to a child. Dads, however, have the highest stature in a child's life, both sons and daughters. For very young children, their first impressions of any male figure are through their dad. He is the standard by which a child judges all other men. For little girls, Dad is their first love, and for little boys, Dad is their first hero.

Several years ago I saw a particular "For Better, For Worse" comic in the newspaper. It was a five-box comic that featured an older man and his grown son leaning on the porch railing, gazing into the night sky. The first two boxes simply show the two men silently gazing. In the third box, the dad says, "I'm proud of you, son. You're doing a good job." In the fourth box, the dad has his hand on his son's shoulder, and the son replies, "Thanks, Dad." In the fifth box, there is a thought bubble over their heads, with both of them thinking the same thing, "Who says men can't have profound personal conversations?" That seems to sum up how the majority of men communicate: a few words, a lot of meaning.

Although it might not look obvious, I'll bet your dad did the best he could. If your dad is here on Earth, make sure you tell him thank you and celebrate what he taught you. Enjoy reminiscing all of the stories, and share the lessons you caught. And tell him that you love him. That's it. I don't need to say much.

His Donation

One of our volunteers, Donna, was assisting at my hospice's annual cookie walk. It is our Christmas fundraiser that involves people buying a typical to-go Styrofoam box for a set donation. The attendees walk along the tables and fill the container with any cookie(s) they like. Each year the event gets bigger to the point where, an hour before this year's event, people started to line up. Did I mention this is in December in Ohio, where it can get pretty cold and snowy?

This year a somewhat disheveled man came in. It was obvious that he had been outside for a while in the falling snow. His shoulders were wet, and his drooping backpack had a slight accumulation of snow on its top flap. He had never been to the event before and asked what was going on. After being told it was a fundraiser to assist the terminally ill and their families, he pulled out his wallet and placed a $10 bill in the donation container.

Then he went into the main room and saw all the cookies and crafts. He couldn't believe the incredible selection of homemade cookies and the variety of crafts. After much thought, he selected just a few cookies' worth, only about one dollar, and approached the checkout table. After a little small talk about the weather, one of our volunteers, Donna, asked the man if he wanted to be on our mailing list. He declined, saying that his address might change since he was staying at the homeless shelter.

Hearing that, and realizing he had spent ten times more on others than he had on himself, Donna said, "We gave him hot coffee and a bag of doughnuts to take with him. He told us he'd share them with those at the shelter."

Whatever caused him to live in a shelter was irrelevant. The fact was the homeless man gave ten times more to others than he kept for himself. And the "others" were people he would never meet, those under hospice care. His donation was truly a gift, and in reality was a lesson of love and caring. Someone who had nothing gave everything.

February is Heart Month

WE HEAR A lot about February being Heart Month, with the emphasis being on our heart's physical health. But everyone knows there are many definitions and interpretations for the word "heart." The primary definition is a noun describing the vital organ that pumps our blood. Or you may hear it called the "ticker" by some. All other definitions of the word "heart" are expressed more as feelings and emotions. That's where hospice's heart is centered. It's what is within those invisible "hearts" that truly gives our life meaning.

Hospice is perceived to be, at least on the surface, a medical organization dealing with any life-limiting illnesses or incurable diseases, including those of the heart. The fact is we are vastly different from other types of medical specialties in that our focus is on the person's emotional and spiritual needs as much as, if not more so than an individual's physical needs. We use a more holistic approach to care.

People who have experienced our level of compassion understand that we have a heart for what we do. One recent afternoon, a family member of someone on our service asked, "What does the application for employment at hospice ask you? All of the staff here have such big hearts. How do you find them?"

Obviously, she wasn't talking about our tickers in the physical sense. She was touching on the definition of heart relating to empathy. I want to share a short story now that really gets to the "heart" of the matter. This story illustrates how a simple gesture by two of our aides speaks volumes about the heart of hospice.

Ruthie, the daughter-in-law of a woman on our hospice, was

awakened at 2:45 a.m. by a phone call from the Pickering House nurse. Ruthie's mother-in-law appeared to be approaching her final hour, and the nurse recommended any family members who wanted should come immediately to be with her. Several days earlier Ruthie's mother-in-law had been brought to the Pickering House for end-of-life care. Since that time, the family had kept a vigil at her bedside.

No one had gotten much sleep during the last few days as it had seemed as if the woman was very close to the end. Even though they had been offered overnight accommodations at the Pickering House, the family decided to go home for some physical as well as emotional rest that evening.

Following the phone call, Ruthie and her family rushed to get there as soon as they could. They didn't want the matriarch of the family to die alone. The family arrived at 4:40 a.m., filled with foreboding. The apprehension, the anxiety, the surreal-like numbness of what was happening made Ruthie feel as it were somehow a dream. What a comfort it was to their family when the nurse met them as they entered the Pickering House.

The nurse walked with them down the now-familiar hall. As she opened the door to the mother-in-law's room, there was a stillness that was hard to define. The room was dimly lit, quiet, and had a spiritual feeling about it. The outside world ceased to exist.

Ruthie and her husband hesitantly entered the room. Startled, Ruthie noticed two women sitting at her mother-in-law's bedside, one on each side of the bed. She quickly recognized them as Pickering House aides. Gently touching Ruthie's hand as they got up to leave, one of the aides whispered, "We didn't want her to be alone." Thirty minutes later, Ruthie's mother-in-law died.

Ruthie later shared, "What a comfort it was to have these two angels, who barely knew us, decide on their own to sit with my mother-in-law until we arrived. I now understand that, yes, hospice's staff, all of their staff, really do care about those under their care."

Now when you hear of February being Heart Month, I hope you think of it a little differently. Understand that your emotional heart health is as important as your physical heart health. Rest assured knowing that during the last stage of life, hospice will focus on your emotional heart health when your physical heart is ready to let go.

Celebrate Independence

THE FOURTH OF July holiday was originally known as Independence Day, for it was on July 4, 1776, that the colonies ratified the Declaration of Independence. "Independence" may be defined as self-rule or self-sufficient, with these definitions applying to either a country or a person. We all know people who are independent. That is, they don't want others to tell them what they should or shouldn't do. That is exactly what we do at hospice—we give those on our service independence.

When someone signs onto our service, the person's plan of care is developed around the question, "What does the patient want?" After all of the months or years of having life ruled by disease, we throw off the shackles of treatments, restricted diets, medicine side effects, and countless trips to medical facilities. We allow people, if they are able, to decide how and where they want to spend this time in their life.

Several years ago a man I'll call "Marty" signed onto my hospice's service. He was in his forties and had been told by his doctor that he had cancer. His doctor told him, with aggressive treatment, he would most likely have eight months of life remaining.

"How long would I live without treatment?" he asked.

"Without treatment? Are you nuts?" was the doctor's reply, according to Marty.

Marty was single, a veteran, and loved his Harley-Davidson motorcycle. And yes, he was serious about no treatment. He just wanted to keep living until he couldn't. Marty was a classic example of someone who didn't want to spend his last months on Earth trying not to die.

Since Marty was so young, his doctor would not refer him

to hospice. That was okay because Marty left the doctor's office and, according to his story, he "found one who would recommend hospice for him."

As we do with every new person, our social worker asked questions about Marty's likes, hobbies, regrets, and anything else to help us truly understand who he was. The social worker found out in no time that Marty liked to "run his own railroad," as my dad used to say.

Marty knew hospice was there to comfort his pain if he had any. If he didn't want comfort medications, that was okay with us. The only rule established was that he would not ride his Harley if he took any pain medicine because the medicine could make him drowsy.

Our hospice team's granting his independence certainly made visiting Marty interesting. No one ever knew if he would be home or not for his weekly scheduled visit. If he felt like riding, well, he did. He wasn't about to ask anyone's permission to ride his own motorcycle. This independent lifestyle was the perfect way for him to live out his life. After all, that was the way he'd lived his whole life, and he didn't want to stop now.

His continuation of life as usual might be one of the reasons Marty lived much longer than his doctor estimated. Per Medicare guidelines, his health was reviewed by a physician every ninety days for his first six months, then every thirty days after that. He continued to decline in health, thus remaining hospice appropriate.

Almost a year after Marty initially signed on, he was asked by the hospice volunteer coordinator if he wanted to join the volunteers as our guest of honor in the approaching Fourth of July parade. He did, and wow, did he have fun! One of the volunteers had already made arraignments to have a 1962 Chrysler Imperial four-door as our parade vehicle. It was almost large enough to call it our float. Marty was riding in style. At one point during the parade, so many of his friends ran out to get their picture with him sitting in the car that the parade came to a brief halt.

When someone accepts our care during what is expected to be the last stage of life (defined by Medicare as six months or less), the person should be free to eat, drink, and be merry all that he or she wants. People are free to celebrate their independence, tie up all the loose ends of their past (*and a few parades*), and enjoy a pain-free life. Many hospices offer this entirely at no cost! Isn't that something worth celebrating?

The County Fair

I LOVE THE COUNTY fair. One of the things that makes the fair so important to me is the reassurance that no matter what goes on in my life, the annual fair is coming. In the three-county service area of my hospice, the first is the Perry County Fair in July, followed by the Hocking County Fair in September, and rounding out the season is the Fairfield County Fair in October. They serve as mile markers as the year moves along. That consistency, like the mail carrier stopping by every day, helps keep my life in order.

As a little boy, my first memories of the fair involve cotton candy; I loved it. However, I soon found out the only place I could get cotton candy was at the fair. Another early memory was Mom saying, "Oh my, look at those prices! We'll buy just one and share."

The fair evolves yet stays the same. Young 4-Hers grow up to be 4-H judges. Cars that I remember as new are now in the Demolition Derby, and the kids on the rides will someday bring their grandchildren to the fair. The truck and tractor pull will always be on Saturday night, and the "Attention on the Midway!" public address announcements will never be replaced by email blasts (I hope). All of these things give me a secure feeling in a life of constant change and turmoil.

So many on hospice service have fond memories of their county fair, and like me, these memories sometimes deal with the high prices. As a patient-contact volunteer, one of the people I would visit told me that when he was a child during the Great Depression, his family would eat dinner before they went to the fair in the evening. He remembered all of the bright lights and the excitement. As he grew up, the man realized that his mother fixed a big dinner before they went so that he and his siblings wouldn't be begging for fair food. Of course, they did anyway! So while at the fair, his siblings would each get a box of Cracker Jacks. The man recalled that the boxes were bigger back then.

Last September, Linda, our in-patient facility's cook, came into my office and asked if she could have a pass to go to the fair. Why? She wanted the pass because she had been reminiscing with one of those staying in the facility about the Hocking County Fair that was in progress. While talking, the subject of fair food came up. Around here, that's all it takes.

Linda came in, asked for, and received a pass. She was soon on her way off to the fair to pick up the two items the patient had been dreaming about: Italian sausage with onions and peppers, and those infamous sugar waffles covered with powdered sugar. I know Linda would have gone to get the food even if the passes hadn't been available.

When Linda returned, the man was overjoyed to see and smell such special food. Even though he technically couldn't eat the food, one of our Pickering House STNAs put just a dab of the juices from the sandwich on his tongue. After he savored the sensation for a few heavenly moments, the STNA placed a touch of powdered sugar on his lips so he could lick it off.

Is fair food good for a hospice patient? (Is it really good for anybody?) That is not a question of importance to us. Who cares what's "good for you" in the last stage of life? It is simply a matter of if the person wants it, the person gets it.

On a more serious note, if someone who loved to go to the fair with you died during the past year, it's going to be a completely different fair experience this time. Nothing will be the same, yet it will all be the same. If you're thinking about going to the fair, my suggestion is to go ahead and go. Consider going with someone who has also suffered a loss. Visit the places that bring back memories. Support each other as you share the good memories that a booth, a ride, or a certain building evoke.

While there, it's okay to cry. It is good to cry and then laugh and rejoice in the moment.

The fair isn't just about 4H and fried food. It's also about happy memories and emotional food. It is about everything that is good in life. Everything is going to be okay. The fair is coming!

Christmas Angels

With all the seasonal hoopla about Black Friday, Small Business Saturday, Cyber Monday, and Giving Tuesday leading up to Christmas, how about an Angel Wings Wednesday? After all, it was an angel who announced to Mary that she was with child that set the stage for the Christmas story. Perhaps remembering that angel would help put some spirituality back into the season.

Maybe on Angel Wings Wednesday we could use the day to thank all of the undercover angels who surround us in our daily lives. I've been told many angels work in the health-care field of hospice. I say this because many of the thank-you cards we receive at my hospice thank the "angels" who cared for their family members.

Looking over the thank-you cards, I've noticed many families have referred to our nursing staff and aides as angels who, as one person wrote, "quietly came into our house and replaced our fear with calmness." Others have thanked us for our hospice aides, who were described as "Christmas angels who decorated our mom's Pickering House room with a Christmas tree and presents months before Christmas. She was so happy to see that." Some thank-you cards have mentioned our angels allowed them rest and moments of peace and serenity, making a bad situation "as good as it could be." One person wrote, "She wiped my tears and shared her own. "

Yes, angels are among us, but I doubt "Angel Wings Wednesday" will catch on. Look for the angels in your life, not only during the hectic Christmas season, but every day.

Attention on the Midway

I LOVE ALL OF the area county fairs. Each one has its own feel. But I don't think any of the fairs have the feel of our Fairfield County Fair. At the fair, there is the heartening consistency of "that's the way we've always done it," while giving a nod to improving a few things here and there. It is one of those comforting annual rituals of life that brings reassurance and tells me that no matter how things have changed, the Fairfield County Fair will always be the second week in October. Yes, everything is going to be okay.

FAIRHOPE Hospice and Palliative Care, Inc. became involved with the fair soon after our agency was formed right here in Fairfield County in 1984. For years, we set up a small display in the art hall at the fair. Now we are found every year in a larger booth on the south end of the same building.

For me, the best part of being at our display is hearing the wondrous stories from people who have experienced our care and compassion. While at our booth, I hear so many stories of how our aides, STNAs, nurses, social workers, chaplains, and volunteers have comforted people. They tend to mention those thoughtful kindnesses no one else would ever think about, yet no one ever forgets. In fact, some of the articles that I have written are the result of those conversations.

If you see a hospice booth at your county fair or any public gathering, why not stop by and say hi?

Giving Your Heart to Another

FEBRUARY IS KNOWN nationally as Heart Month. The term "Heart Month" spurred me to think of what I've learned at hospice concerning giving your heart to someone else. I have been fortunate enough to witness quite a few married couples whose final wedding vow, "Til death do us part," becomes fulfilled. It is fascinating and insightful to become acquainted with couples who have been together for the majority of their lives. My own unscientific observations have revealed that lifelong marriages generally result in much fewer regrets at the end of life.

When discussing marriage with these couples, the question of the secret to a long marriage invariably comes up. In one particular instance, the husband of a woman on our hospice gave an answer I had never heard before. He said that he had to realize early on that his wife was a person just as he was a person, shortcomings and all.

As he and I continued our conversation, he recalled when they first fell in love, she seemed to be perfect. Therefore, after their wedding, he expected her to continue to be perfect. He had the insight to realize even though he thought he was accepting of her "defects of character" (as he sheepishly told me), they were, in essence, only being ignored. Honestly accepting his wife as she actually was made him fall into a true, deep love for her.

As it turned out, the man and I had very similar expectations and results. From my perspective, when I said, "I do," I thought my wife, Vickie, was perfect and would always be that way. To be honest, I was wrong in a few areas. But as this man did, I (subconsciously) began to recognize my wife's differences.

After over forty-eight years of marriage, I have a deep love for her and am so thankful for our life together.

This conversation occurred during February. We had brought his wife to my hospice's in-patient facility, the Pickering House, for a few-day stay in order to manage the symptoms of her disease. One of our aides told me she noticed how the man held his wife's hand as our staff was getting the newly arrived woman settled in her bed.

After the woman was situated, she mentioned almost casually how she and her husband used to lie in bed together, hold hands, and watch TV once the kids had grown and moved out. Immediately, the aide asked the husband if he wanted to lie with his wife and watch TV. Caught off guard, the husband stammered when replying yes. He desperately wanted to.

Quickly, our staff got together and assisted the husband to be in bed with his wife. You see, they were fully aware the couple's wedding vow to each other of "Till death do us part" was close to being fulfilled. Our remarkable hospice staff knows at this stage of life, accompaniment, not technology, may be the most caring thing we can offer.

Once her husband gently cuddled next to her, the woman leaned her head against his shoulder; their fingers entwined. They could feel each other's warmth. All the couple needed was to be together, alone. Our staff turned on the couple's favorite TV show, dimmed the room lights, and after a short gaze, left.

Yes, the roses, the heart-shaped box of candy, and romantic dinners all get the attention when talking about giving your heart to another. Those are physical things. As life progresses, the importance of the small acts we do that may not always be seen takes precedence. Helen Keller fully understood this when she said, "The best and most beautiful things in this world cannot be seen or even heard, but must be felt with the heart."

Understanding these invisible emotions, feelings, and attitudes is the "heart" of what we do in hospice.

Military Pinning Service

Part of the admission process for hospice is to get to know the people being admitted and their families. If we are told that a person was a veteran, we will ask if he or she would like to talk about his or her experience. Some do, some don't. Sometimes, even if people are not willing to talk about their experiences, we mindfully ask if they would like to be thanked for their commitment to our country with a military pinning service. No matter their experience, the answer is usually yes. This service is conducted where the veteran lives, be it in a facility or the person's home.

I spoke to a group several months ago, telling them of the pinning service, and a woman told me that our hospice had performed the service for her dad. She said those in attendance at the pinning, besides her, were our social worker and one of our patient-contact volunteers, who himself was a veteran. She said when her dad was admitted to our service, a pinning was scheduled for a week later, but as his condition worsened, she called to see if it could be performed as soon as possible.

It was late evening, but indications were that the veteran might not have too much longer to live, so now was the time. Understanding the circumstances, the on-call nurse arranged for it immediately. In the darkness, one of our social workers and a military veteran volunteer read the proclamation to thank the man for his service, pinned him on his pajamas' lapel, and presented him with a certificate of appreciation. The volunteer then took a step back and saluted the veteran. The dad, who the daughter thought was in a deep sleep, lifted his right hand with fingers straightened as far as he could to return the salute. The daughter started to cry as she told the story, and to be honest, so did I.

The military pinning is not an award but a recognition of sacrifice. It is a very simple service consisting of reading a proclamation, pinning an American flag pin on the lapel, followed by the branch of service pin below it. This little ceremony is so simple yet so profound. There have been tears or sniffles at every one of the pinnings I have attended. And talk about variety. The services I've attended have ranged from commencing with the entrance of bagpipes to only one family member and a hospice employee very late in the evening. From an elderly man who still fit in his uniform to those wearing the last piece of clothing they would ever wear. From those still able to stand at attention to several who passed before we arrived. In the last scenario, each family requested the honorarium service be conducted, regardless. One pinning was performed during calling hours at the funeral home.

The significance of the service, I believe, is that it recognizes the person is still alive. Attention is being focused on the individual and his or her life, not the person's current condition. It also recognizes the sacrifices the veterans made during life and thanking them for it. All of which are hallmarks of hospice compassion.

Veterans and Their Families

I HAVE EXPERIENCED A lot of Veteran's Days in my life. Veteran's Day acknowledges that any time spent in military service involves sacrifice. Not only do the veterans make sacrifices to be in the military, but often their families have to make sacrifices and adjustments as well, especially if a spouse and children were involved.

Growing up in Fairborn, Ohio, which wraps around the eastern side of Wright-Patterson Air Force Base, I witnessed a little bit of how military service involved the whole family. Many of my neighborhood friends and my classmates had fathers that were in the Air Force. Every September, when school started, approximately a third of my classmates were gone, and there were a bunch of new kids. The reason being , the Air Force tended to transfer most officers every three years, and summer was when the majority of families moved.

I couldn't imagine moving to a new state every three years. Some of my friends had been to different countries; some had been in the desert while at Edwards Air Force Base; and one of my friends in fourth grade had lived in Alaska, Louisiana, and now, Ohio. None of my friends said they enjoyed it, but it was the only life they knew.

That made me start thinking about how on Veteran's Day we honor the people who served in the military, and it is justly deserved. But I would like to briefly discuss how the veterans' service may have temporarily changed the family dynamics and had an influence on all aspects of society.

My dad was of German descent. He was fluent in German and English, and both were spoken in his house while growing up. During WWII, he arrived in France a few weeks after the Normandy invasion. He served in an engineer combat company under Patton in the Low Countries and in Germany. Because of his fluency in German, he served as an interpreter in any situation involving the German military or civilian population and his company.

I've read that the war influenced the generation that fought and the generation that followed. During my parents' generation, the whole country was involved in the war, whether it was in the military, in war production, or living with almost everything being rationed. My generation was the one that followed. I felt the military's influence in everyday life. In Cub Scouts and Boy Scouts, we had uniform inspections. We marched in step in a parade. At home, when the babysitter came over because Mom and Dad were going out for the evening, Dad would call all six of us kids to the living room with an authoritative "front and center." He would then tell us in no uncertain terms that the babysitter was in charge. He was following the military tradition of transferring authority from one "commander" to another with everyone present. There was no misunderstanding that the babysitter was in charge. However, we also knew if she did something against what we knew wasn't right, we should tell him or Mom when they returned.

The Scout Master of my Boy Scout troop was a WWII veteran. In the regular Scout meetings, we wore full uniforms. For parades and other important events, we polished our shoes and would have a full inspection. These are small examples of how the military experience of the previous generation trickled into the next generation. Granted, these examples weren't the traumatic events some of my classmates and friends experienced when their combat-weary fathers came home. But WWII subtly affected nearly everyone in my generation, in one way or another.

The aftereffects of military service may influence veterans

and their families in some unexpected ways. For example, my brother-in-law's dad always kept the refrigerator full and plenty of food in the pantry. I found out years later that he had been a prisoner of war in a German prison camp. His dad said that since that experience of prolonged hunger, he didn't want to take the chance of ever being without food again.

That was a subtle effect of military service, while on the other side of the coin, for some, the effects of military service weren't subtle. As a patient-contact volunteer, one of the assignments I accepted was a veteran of Iwo Jima, a small island in the South Pacific. My volunteer supervisor told me before I accepted the assignment that the man could be sullen or sometimes angry. His wife said he'd been like that since the war. It seemed like sixty years was a long time to still have "shell shock," as PTSD was called after WWII.

During my initial visit, I asked the man about Iwo. He just repeated, "Bad place, bad place." That was the only verbal exchange I had with him.

This assignment was while I was a leasing agent, years before I became a hospice employee. Since I was employed elsewhere, when the man died I took off work because the only visiting hours were from two to four on a Wednesday afternoon. I usually didn't mix work with hospice, but I knew the man's wife needed support.

When I arrived around 3:00 p.m., the parking lot was empty. I thought I had come on the wrong day, which isn't unusual for me. I parked my car and walked to the funeral home door to inquire about when visiting hours were scheduled. I jumped as the door was suddenly opened by an employee. I told him that I must have the wrong day. I asked about the man's calling hours, and he said it was down the hall on the left. Surprised, I walked down the silent, empty hall and went into a large empty room on my left.

There, to the left, was the man's wife standing at the foot of her husband's casket. She said I was the first visitor. My heart sank. I was so grateful that I went. I couldn't imagine that no one had come, not even his family. I just couldn't imagine. But he had brought that "bad place" home with him so many years ago and scared family and friends away.

Even though I have focused on WWII, I have not forgotten Korea, Vietnam, and all of the more recent military conflicts. These also have left their mark on the families of veterans. Whether in combat or not, veterans took time out of their lives to serve, disrupting their family life in the process. During the initial consult, when we learn of someone's military service, we ask if the person would like to talk about his or her service. Some do, and some don't. Usually a family member will. And each family has its own unique story to share to give us an insight into just what sacrifices have been made in service to military and country.

The Simple Act of Showing Up

I GO TO THE visitation or funeral service of each of the people I've been assigned as a patient-contact volunteer. Starting with the first family to whom I was assigned, I'll bet at every service I've attended, I have received a very warm thank you from family members. They thank me for coming to their house and staying with their loved one in order to allow them to take a break from the constant caregiving.

Very quickly, I realized that the people thanking me weren't just being polite. They were, in fact, sincerely appreciative that I would come to their home in order to give them a break from tending to their loved one. Why they wanted to leave for those few hours is not important. Maybe they needed to run errands, go to church, or just leave to take a walk. My experience has been that when someone becomes very ill or terminally ill, most family and friends tend to stay away. The hospice patient-contact volunteer, however, comes in offering assistance.

Thinking back to the first man I visited, I didn't do anything special. He lived in a long-term care facility and was comatose. However, in hospice, even if a person is in a coma and does not respond, we treat the individual as if he or she can still hear. The man's wife wanted me to visit on Tuesday and Thursday evenings and suggested I read to him. I wasn't sure what to read, so I brought in a binder that had a large collection of jokes I'd heard and written down over the years. I believe it brought joy to the man because he made a few slight movements during my visit.

Being a part of hospice, I've learned you never know who you will have an effect on, whether you impact the one who is ill or the person's family. I do know that you won't have an effect on anyone without the simple act of showing up.

Burnt Cheeks

Hospice is in the family business. As both a patient-contact volunteer and a Community Educator, I've heard many family stories over the years. Even as adults, when children talk about their father, many still refer to him as "Daddy." Most of the daddy and father stories tend to be about the life lessons a man taught.

Dads such as mine taught many lessons both by example and by allowing mistakes to be made. I remember when I grew up, playgrounds had steel slides. Not only that, but there were boards on long chains for swings, and the entire play area was covered with gravel. When we'd go to the playground, Dad would tell us only once to be careful. If we fell, he'd clean off any cut and give us a hug. If it was a sunny day and we burned our "cheeks" on the hot metal slide, he'd ask us why we went down it if it was hot.

Life can be similar. If we can see that a certain activity may cause physical or spiritual pain, then we shouldn't do it. But would we want to miss out on this life experience and what it could teach us? Telling me to slow down, not to jump off that, etc., would not have taught me anything. A pair of burnt cheeks is a lesson I've kept with me all of my life.

Yes, we need to be nurtured. But dads like mine tend to use very few words to teach valuable life lessons. I remember when my friends worried that they were turning into their dads; all the while, I tried my best to do just that. Thank you, Dad.

Whether it is Father's Day or just another day in the year, tell your dad thank you for the little things that he did. You won't have to say too much.

A Grilled Cheese Sandwich

A GRILLED CHEESE SANDWICH?! My hospice receives a volume of thank-you cards on a weekly basis. A few months ago, one card in particular mentioned how nice it was that we had prepared a grilled cheese sandwich for her mom. After all the family had gone through, this person was thanking us for a grilled cheese sandwich? The fact that the woman who mailed the thank-you card even mentioned it speaks volumes about the importance of food at the end of life.

I was giving a small group tour of the Pickering House not too long ago. During that tour, I mentioned that in the steady stream of thank-you cards, writers will often pick out a few people or kind gestures that impressed them. I told them about that particular card in which the daughter mentioned how our staff fixed her mom a grilled cheese sandwich. "One of my mom's favorite things. SO NICE!!" she had written. What surprised one person in the group was the idea that we even have a kitchen in the building. Aren't people residing in a hospice facility in the last days of their life?

Looking back, I don't think the person I was talking to believed that the family of someone who was cared for by hospice would remember a gesture as insignificant as a grilled cheese sandwich. In this case I don't know if the woman who received the sandwich could eat it or not; that detail is unimportant and at the same time of absolute importance. The kind gesture made the woman's mom so happy. It touched the heart of her daughter to the point she felt the need to specifically mention it in her thank-you card, and years later at that. She didn't mail the card until several years after her mom was on our service.

After all of the apprehension, fear, sadness, and tension that come with a parent enduring a chronic illness, the daughter remembered a simple, kind gesture. That sums up what hospice is about: understanding the importance of the little things. Every employee in my hospice is empowered to act upon the seemingly casual desires of those at the end of life.

A grilled cheese sandwich sounds relatively common. However, my hospice staff recognized its importance and responded. Hospice is here to enhance someone's life. And in life, it is simple acts of kindness during a time of stress that demonstrate the inherent good of life to the very end.

And Palliative Care

Many hospices in the United States have the words "and Palliative Care" in their name. That is the part of a hospice's name in the United States that describes a very important part of what a hospice organization can do. The palliative care team and the hospice team are two separate entities in the same organization. It is very important to understand that "palliative care" in many parts of the world is hospice care. In the United States, palliative care allows continued treatment of the primary illness.

Palliative (pal-ee-uh-tiv) care might be summed up as care without curing. As mentioned, in the United States, palliative care is a form of medical attention that allows curative treatment to continue. What palliative care contributes is a relief of the symptoms and the emotional stress of a serious illness. Its goal is to give ill people *and their families* the best possible quality of life.

As with hospice, palliative care is provided where the ill person lives. And, as with everything hospice does, most consults to discuss palliative care take place wherever the family wants. The initial consult may take place where the person lives—a home, an apartment, an assisted living community or nursing home. It may also take place in "neutral territory," such as a restaurant.

When discussing palliative care, it is important to note that the physician is still your primary medical contact. The palliative care nurse serves as a liaison between you and your doctor. One of the ways we assist the primary doctor is to keep him or her aware of all aspects of their patient on service. We also may make recommendations to the primary doctor, but they are only recommendations. When you choose to retain your family doctor, the palliative care nurse may consult with your family doctor, just as any specialist would do.

Any chronic illness may qualify for palliative care. As a general guide, the following diagnoses are commonly treated by palliative care: chronic pain, liver disease, dementia, kidney disease, cancer, COPD, lung disease, Parkinson's, and heart disease. There are no restrictions regarding length of care.

The hallmark of hospice is to serve. The focus of care not only includes the person on service and his or her family, but any family pets, should they be a part of the household. Including pets is important not only to the family but for the pet, as well. Pets understand there is a crisis going on and may also be upset due to the influx of visitors. One of our nurses, Billie, told me she always kept dog and cat treats with her to make sure the pet received some attention. I have no doubt she would include fish food if the family had a goldfish.

One of the subtle ways a hospice may provide much-needed emotional support is by the mere act of showing up. Our presence in the home affords emotional and spiritual support at a time when the focus is mainly on the physical aspect of the disease. Many times the person who accepted palliative care lives alone and is lonely. Billie also mentioned to me that as part of her visit, she will sit down and talk to the person for a half hour or so. For most on service, visits by our palliative nurse are an anticipated event. Besides our nursing staff, social workers and chaplains are also available with palliative care to give support when difficult medical decisions need to be made.

Life has its burdens. The constant worry when dealing with a serious illness is a burden that can easily prevent life from being enjoyed. When confronted with such a situation, a measure of peace can be achieved when your doctor and palliative care work together.

Enjoyable and Satisfying

Every hospice is blessed to have a wonderful group of volunteers. All hospice volunteers are vital to ensure that hospice fulfills its mission of helping those under their care. Hospice came into existence through the efforts of volunteers, but they aren't just a luxury. Medicare requires at least 5 percent of all hospice patient-care hours be provided by volunteers.

Hospice volunteers fulfill many roles. Sometimes they assist in the business office. Some help with fundraising, while many are patient-contact volunteers or reach out to families through bereavement support calls. Volunteers choose in what area they want to serve. At my hospice, it may be all four.

Of the four areas of volunteering, the patient-contact volunteer is offered several unique privileges. The patient-contact volunteer is given the privilege of entering into someone's life to help a person complete goals and relive special delights in his or her personal history.

Will Rogers said, "We all can't be heroes. Someone has to sit on the curb and clap as they go by." The volunteer allows the person on service to be the star of the show by allowing the individual to recount his or her successes, failures, funny stories, regrets, accomplishments, and goals.

Supporting someone on our hospice with his or her goals may involve helping the person reunite with an estranged child. It may be connecting the individual with people to help him or her complete a train layout as a final gift to a grandson. Or it may be lending a hand to a Marine veteran whose goal is to put his fishing boat away for the winter so that everything is in order and he can die in peace. Completing personal goals is an important part of the final stage of life. Patient-contact volunteers are often involved in helping make these final requests possible.

Along those lines, the patient-contact volunteer is in the position to help people relive a favorite activity one final time. For example, one of our volunteers, Margie, was talking to a woman, Kay, who was staying for a few days at our hospice facility, Pickering House. She was lamenting about how all her life she loved going on picnics. Sadly, now that she was ill and bedridden, Kay knew she would never go on another picnic.

On her way home, Margie thought, "Why not bring a picnic to Kay?" The next day the two of them shared a lovely picnic on the woman's bed in the Pickering House. It was that simple. The woman said the only thing missing was the ants.

As with Margie, many of the activities in which patient-contact volunteers are involved consist of a one-last-time event. Over twenty years ago, as a patient-contact volunteer, I was visiting with a man while his wife went shopping. When I arrived, he was sitting in his favorite chair, a recliner. After his wife left, the man decided he wanted to nap, so he slowly got up out of the recliner. His bed was a mere five feet away. I helped him get out of his recliner and waited while he steadied his feet. I assisted him by holding his arm as he took the short walk to his bed.

As it turned out, I walked with the man during the last steps he ever took. The volunteer coordinator called me the next day and said the man's kidneys had begun to shut down. He died two days later. I got to thinking that over eighty years ago, the man had taken his first step, most likely with a lot of fanfare from his parents. I had the honor to be with him when he took his last steps after all of those millions of steps throughout his life.

I frequently hear comments about how sad it must be to volunteer for a hospice. Whether at a hospice in-patient facility or in the home of someone on hospice, our volunteers help people celebrate and complete their lives. As far as I am concerned, there is nothing more enjoyable and satisfying than that.

The Camel

I DON'T THINK THERE is an area of life where prayer is more intense, more fervent, than during the last stage. As life ebbs, the physical and emotional aspects of life fade, and all that remains is the spiritual realm. Cognitive of the significant need for spiritual comfort, hospice includes the spiritual needs of the one contemplating our care. During the initial consult, the person or family member is asked about his or her spiritual belief system. The purpose of the inquiry regarding the individual's spiritual condition is the same as when inquiring about his or her physical and emotional status. It helps us learn as much about the person as the individual wants to divulge. Our plan of care is formed around the whole person, not the disease.

Spirituality is an area of discussion that must be considered when contemplating which hospice to call. Some organizations may favor one belief system over another. Most hospices, including mine, have only one requirement for acceptance. That is, the primary physician feels that if the disease progresses at its normal rate, the patient has six months or less of life remaining. Notice the statement does not include spiritual beliefs and has no mention of religious denomination. "Six months or less of life remaining" is what makes a person eligible for hospice care. The freedom to discuss spirituality or decline any questions in regard to addressing the spiritual aspect of the last stage of life is always present.

Within the family, there can be discussions concerning why God gives us such a burden. I have heard that question answered two different ways. The most common answer is that God doesn't give us more than we can handle. The second answer I have heard, especially from pastors, is that God does give us more than we can handle so that we rely on God to get us through. The vast majority of hospices don't enter that discussion. But no matter what you believe, it is certain that a burden will be carried, and prayer will be frequent.

I have heard prayer described in many ways. During times of trouble, one way that makes sense to me is thinking about the camel in the desert regions of North Africa and Arabia. Camels have been the main means of long-distance travel since biblical times. In a caravan, camels would kneel down in the evening, and the men would unload the camels' burdens. In the morning, the camels would kneel down again, and the men would put the burdens back on.

For me, that it is the same analogy with prayer. I get on my knees at night and ask God to unload my burdens. Then each morning, I get on my knees again. Normally, God gives me just the load I am able to carry for that day. But sometimes, as I mentioned above, I need to lean on Him.

Every hospice will work to determine what brings those under its care spiritual comfort and assist as best it can. As with the camel, hospice strives to remove the day's burdens so that life may be lived in comfort and peace.

What Does a Nursing Assistant Do?

I HAVE BEEN A patient-contact volunteer for over twenty-four years. During so many of my visits, when the spouse is preparing to leave, she will give her husband (who is on our hospice) the shortlist of hospice staff who may be stopping by. Experience has shown me the most important person expected to visit is no surprise. It is the man or woman who is the nursing assistant.

Being in the forefront as a somewhat passive observer to hospice, I have learned much about everyday hospice care. A good percentage of what I have learned is not so much what is in the books and brochures about *amazing care* by *amazing staff*; rather it is about what is most important to the person receiving the care. Not only is the person receiving a great deal of attention, but so is the family. To see so much attention focused on a loved one gives the family assurance that they are not alone.

Each hospice generally assigns a registered nurse (RN); possibly a licensed practical nurse (LPN), also known as a licensed vocational nurse (LVN); a nursing assistant (aide, CNA, STNA); a social worker; and the offer of a chaplain and a volunteer to be of assistance. The one who makes the most favorable impression, by my unscientific study, is the nursing assistant. Theirs is a title that varies by region: nurse aide, certified nurse aide (CNA), nursing assistant, certified nurse assistant (CNA), patient care assistant (PCA), and state-tested nursing assistant (STNA). I'm sure that I have left a few titles out, but at the core they are the angels of hospice care. Probably the easiest way to describe what they do is to use the short version of the Prayer of St. Francis. It follows:

> Lord, make me an instrument of Your Peace: where there is hatred, let me sow love. Where there is doubt, faith, where there is despair, hope. Where there is darkness, light. Where there is sadness, joy.
>
> O Divine Master, grant that I may not so much seek to be consoled as to console; to be understood as to understand; to be loved, as to love; for it is in giving that we receive, it is in pardoning that we are pardoned, and it is in dying that we are born to eternal life.

Let's take a look at that prayer line by line, from the perspective of a nursing assistant:

Where there is hatred, let me sow love. Since the late 1990s, I am aware of only two people with AIDS who have been under the care of my hospice's service. Both of the people, by their own admission, had become infected with AIDS as a result of their lifestyle. And they felt they were now paying the price.

However, their parents were also paying the price, although they had done nothing to deserve it. The parents heard derogatory comments about AIDS patients wherever they went. They hurt because their sons were suffering and because no one seemed to care about them.

No one cared until the families called my hospice and our staff entered their lives. I remember when one of our STNAs gently, tenderly put salve on one of the men's sores. I felt as if I was watching Mother Teresa. The STNA told me she only sees the need, not the cause.

Where there is injury, pardon. Our home-side nursing assistants visit the people on hospice wherever they live. In one particular setting, a newly hired nurse assistant had a difficult person she was caring for. After a few months, when the dying process started, the man reached for her arm and, in a barely audible voice, said, "Thank you. I love you." The nursing assistant had taken the brunt of his anger over her previous visits with him. She endured much but understood where it came from. Those five words confirmed that this was where she belonged.

Where there is doubt, faith. People always think of the future, perhaps thinking of an upcoming vacation, a special outing with friends, or simply a day to enjoy one of life's pleasures. When someone becomes terminal, everything changes because the person runs out of future. Doubt begins to settle in rather than looking forward to what lies ahead. Our nurse assistants remove a person's doubt and fear by looking at the individuals with the eyes of faith. By their presence, nurse assistants bring emotional and spiritual comfort to those at the end of their life.

Where there is despair, hope. Often, terminally ill people have been lying in bed for an extended period. Often they may experience depression. The anticipation of the nurse assistant's arrival gives them something to look forward to as a ray of hope.

Where there is darkness, light. I was talking to one of our nurse assistants, Stephanie, and she said that whenever she tells someone she works in hospice, she gets admonished in some fashion. "That's so depressing." "How can you work there? Can't you find something better?" Truth is, Stephanie has been with us for quite a few years, and she told me she wouldn't want to be anywhere else. She lights up the lives of the people on service with her unconditional and empathetic love.

Where there is sadness, joy. A woman was brought to the Pickering House for symptom management. She seemed depressed. Talking to her, one of the nurse assistants discerned that she had been engaged for quite a while, and now it looked like she and her fiancé would never get married. Hearing this, plans were quickly made by the staff of the Pickering House, the in-patient facility of my hospice, and the couple was married that evening. While the ceremony was taking place in the Sun Room, the staff eagerly made the new bride's room into a "honeymoon suite." Through tears of joy, the woman said, "Now I am complete."

Grant that I may not so much seek to be consoled as to console. Patsy, one of our nurse assistants, walked into a person's room to give her a massage. The lady was curled up in a ball, not from pain, but from fear. Over the next hour, as Patsy gave her a slow, gentle massage, she sang and prayed for her. The lady relaxed to the point that Patsy said she would lift the woman's arm a tiny bit, and it would "plop" down on the bed. The woman went to sleep as Patsy was shampooing her hair. When Patsy told me about this, she said it had been a rough day up to that point, but the ill person came first, and Patty came second.

To be understood, as to understand. Near the end of her shift, Carla, a Pickering House nurse assistant, was pushing a man on service in a wheelchair. He had been restless, and she was hopeful this would relax him. The man noticed a woman carrying her purse, a floral arrangement, and a shopping bag. He asked if he could take them to the door for her. "Sure, I could use the help. I hope my purse isn't too big," she said with a laugh. He placed the three items on his lap, and Carla pushed him to the front door, where the woman thanked him. Earlier the man felt that he was "wastin' away," as he put it. Intuitively, Carla understood his need to be needed.

To be loved, as to love. I was talking to a woman whose mother had been on hospice. She mentioned that she had never forgotten how tenderly Kelly, the nurse assistant, would touch her mother. She also mentioned that when her mother wanted to talk, Kelly would pull up a chair and sit next to the bed so that she would be at eye level. "Where do you find people with so much love?" she asked.

It is in giving that we receive. Every nurse assistant I have talked to has told me they receive much more than they give. A family member told me that she was "almost startled" by the cheerfulness of our aides.

It is in pardoning that we are pardoned. Our nurse assistants sometimes may deal with difficult people. It is a part of the job. They understand the emotion of a person losing control of his or her life. They easily pardon any negative emotion because it is not aimed at them.

And it is in dying that we are born to eternal life. Angela, a longtime nurse assistant, told me about a woman she was tending to at an assisted living community. When Angela visited one afternoon, she noticed that the dying process had started.

The woman always had a two-bulb lamp lit next to her bed, but as Angela approached the woman's bed, one of the lights went out. She didn't think too much about it at the time. Sensing that the woman's final hour was approaching, Angela sat at the woman's bedside. At almost the same instant that the woman took her last breath, the second bulb went out. The room was now dim, and Angela was enveloped by the spirituality of the moment. She was there at the most important moment in the woman's life, as she entered eternal life.

What does a nurse assistant do? I think the quickest way to find out is to listen to the words of St. Francis.

Alone No More

I was at my hospice's in-patient facility, the Pickering House, talking to the volunteer manager. We talked for a few minutes, then she asked me if I would relieve a new volunteer who had been sitting for quite a while with someone in a room. The volunteer was sitting at the bedside of a comatose man whose hour was approaching. No visitors had come since his arrival. What was so unusual was the man was younger than the average person on our hospice. People his age tended to have many visitors.

When I entered the room, Pat, my fellow volunteer, was rubbing the man's arm while softly talking to him. I sat in silence with her for a few minutes. She finally broke the silence by saying that as a member of our No One Dies Alone (NODA) program, she was fully aware of the eventual outcome. With emotion in her voice, Pat continued, "But this one is getting to me. It is so sad." The man was disfigured due to his illness and, because of long-standing family problems, had been abandoned by his small family.

Then she expressed how thankful she was to God for leading her to volunteer at a hospice, ultimately guiding her to this man's room on this particular morning. She said she just couldn't imagine him dying by himself, regardless of what his family life had been like.

Her comments struck me as the epitome of love—putting others first. Her comments also demonstrated an understanding of hospice's philosophy that companionship, not technology, may be the most caring thing we can offer those facing death.

Mother Teresa said, "Your true character is accurately

measured by how you treat those who can do nothing for you." Words with great meaning, to be emulated and lived by so that no one dies alone.

CHAPTER 5
When Death Approaches

"One of the subliminal aspects of the hospice philosophy of care is that it gives the opportunity to arrive at the conclusion of life with a genuine sense completion."

The Conclusion of Life

*S*IMPLE *H*UMAN *C*OMPASSION is about the last stage of life. For that reason, it seemed natural to end the book with a general description of what the last days and hours of life entail. This description is a generalization because, as will be noted in the following, each person is unique and so is his or her end-of-life progression. As you read this, keep in mind there is no mention of a need for technology or medical procedures, only compassion and love. The last stage of life is unique unto itself.

As of this writing, I have been associated with hospice for over twenty-four years. I go to the funerals of those I visited as a patient-contact volunteer. At many of the funerals or memorial services, a family member will come up to me and thank me for "that book" given to them when their loved one was admitted to hospice service. That book, actually a simple twelve-page booklet, is included in the informational packet given to every family whose loved one is admitted to my hospice's care.

Each hospice has its own variation of the booklet. To guide the family as they prepare for the approaching event, the members of the hospice care team will help everyone identify the various indicators for each stage of the dying process as it is entered. The knowledge of the end-of-life process offers those close family and friends the chance to comfort their family member gently and lovingly.

So, what makes this booklet so significant and memorable? What the booklet does is describe the dying process in an honest and gentle, but to the point, way. The information allows the caregiver and other family members to understand the physical and mental changes that occur as their loved one enters the last days and hours of life. Importantly, it also explains why these changes occur. It is of tremendous comfort for families to have this knowledge because it gives them a sense of being a part of what is happening rather than being idle bystanders.

A basic insight into the dying process removes some of the apprehension those involved may have as the completion of life approaches. So often I hear from family members that through understanding what is happening, they were able to care for their mother at the end of her life just as she comforted them at the beginning of theirs. What a gift!

Hospice eligibility begins when the prognosis is anticipated to be six months or less of life remaining. Notice that I said "anticipated"? It is not an exact science to determine when a person has entered the last stage of life. To be eligible for the Medicare Hospice Benefit, it is required that either two physicians or one hospice-certified physician believes the ill person has six months or less of life remaining if the disease follows its natural course.

As the person acknowledges—ergo accepts—that he or she is dying, generally with a few months of life remaining, the person may withdraw from normal outside interests. Next, the individual will probably withdraw from people. As the person withdraws, there is less of a need to talk. Words lose their importance, and touch becomes more significant.

When a person enters the final weeks of life, two different dynamics are at work—the physical plane and the emotional-mental-spiritual plane. These dynamics are closely interrelated and interdependent. On the physical plane, the body begins the final process of shutting down, which ends when all the physical systems cease to function. Usually this is an orderly and undramatic progressive series of physical changes, which are not medical emergencies requiring invasive interventions. The most appropriate kinds of responses are comfort-enhancing measures.

During this stage of the physical shutting down, a person will refuse food. The body's rejection of food is a clear indicator that the completion of life is approaching. Since the purpose of food is to sustain life, it is natural for the body to reject it as life is ending. It is also counterintuitive to everything we've known about comforting someone. The rejection of food is by far the hardest transition for all involved to accept.

When the person has only a few days of life remaining, his or her breathing may vary from a breath around every ten to fifteen seconds up to almost a breath a second. The individual's blood pressure lowers, and the skin may feel clammy. The skin color changes, and the hands and feet may develop a pale blue color as the blood circulation diminishes. What may be surprising is that there may be a very noticeable increase in energy, which may include talking to those present. A decrease in oxygen in the blood may make the person restless.

The other dynamic during the last hours of the dying process is the emotional-spiritual-mental plane. Changes occur simultaneously with the physical dynamic. There is a different kind of process in which the "spirit" of the dying person begins the final process of release from the body, its immediate environment, and all attachments. This release also tends to follow its own priorities, which may include the resolution of whatever is unfinished of a practical nature and the reception of permission to "let go" from family members. These events are the normal, natural way in which the spirit prepares to move from this existence into the next dimension of life. The most appropriate kinds of responses to the emotional-spiritual-mental changes are those which support and encourage this release and transition.

When a person's body is ready and wants to stop but the person still has unresolved or unreconciled conflicts over an important issue, or a conflict with some significant relationship, he or she may tend to linger. Although the lingering may be uncomfortable or debilitating, it continues in order to finish whatever needs finishing.

When your loved one is ready to die and you are able to let go, then is the time to say goodbye. This is your final gift of love to your loved one, for it achieves closure and makes the final release possible. It may be helpful to lie in bed with the person and hold him or her. Maybe take the person's hand and then say everything you need to say. It may be as simple as saying, "I love you." It may include recounting favorite memories, places, and activities you shared. It may include saying, "I'm sorry for (fill in what you feel needs to be said)." It may also include saying thank you for any reason important to you.

Tears are a normal and natural part of saying goodbye. Tears do not need to be hidden from your loved one, nor do they need to be apologized for. They express your love and help you to let go.

The experience we call death occurs when the body completes its natural process of shutting down and when the "spirit" completes its natural process of reconciling and finishing. These two processes need to happen in a way that is appropriate and unique to the values, beliefs, and lifestyle of the dying person. In keeping with the fact that the end of life is unique unto itself, the death of someone on hospice service is not an emergency. Hospice will need to be notified, and a nurse will come to your location and help with what needs to be done.

The end of life is not a particularly pleasant topic for most people. However, being aware of what is to come and facing it will help to relieve some of the fear the end of life evokes. Fear will force us to seek and identify choices. I hope the knowledge gained here presents options and allows an agreeable decision to be made.

Glossary

Advance Care Planning - Planning about the care you would want if you could no longer speak for yourself due to an illness.

Advance Directive - A document that describes the types of decisions you should make before you become seriously ill and unable to speak for yourself. This can be done at any age.

Aide – *See nursing assistant.*

Anticipatory Grief - Mourning the death of a loved one before that person has died. This occurs frequently when someone close is terminally ill.

Bereavement – The state of having suffered a loss.

Burnout – exhaustion, anger and depression that develop from feeling alone and unsupported as you care for a loved one.

Calling Hours – Usually held at a funeral home, the body of the diseased is displayed, allowing mourners the opportunity to pay their respects.

Case Manager – Generally the Registered Nurse whose coordination of services is required to care for the terminally ill person.

Chaplain - a clergy or lay person employed by a hospice. A chaplain ministers to those of any religious belief, and of no religious belief. Also see: Spiritual Care Coordinator.

CNA – Certified Nursing Assistant. Also *see nurse aide, nursing assistant, STNA.*

Continuous Care—one of the four levels of care mandated by the Medicare hospice benefit; up to 24 hours/day of clinical care in the home until symptoms are under control.

Curative Care—Treatments intended to cure a disease

Diagnosis—Determination of the disease or condition that explains a person's symptoms or ailments.

Difference between hospice and palliative care—Palliative care is the larger umbrella: all care that is intended to comfort the patient with a serious or chronic illness, not cure the disease. Hospice care is a sub-category of comfort care reserved for terminally ill patients who do not opt for curative treatment.

DNR—a do not resuscitate (DNR) order is written by a physician at the request of a terminally ill patient and placed in the patient's records. It instructs medical staff not to revive the patient if their breathing or heartbeat stops.

Dysphagia - difficulty swallowing

Dyspnea - difficult or labored breathing

Edema - an excess of fluid in body cavities or beneath the skin. It causes swelling and is very painful.

Election of Hospice – The decision to accept hospice and signing of the necessary paperwork.

End-of-life - (e-o-l) care - see hospice care.

Family Caregiver – A family member who provides physical and/or emotional care to the terminally ill family member at home.

Four Levels of Care - the Medicare hospice benefit mandates that a hospice offer four levels of care to qualify for Medicare reimbursement. Those levels are: routine home care, continuous care, general inpatient care (GIP) and respite care. See Continuous Care, General Inpatient (GIP) Care, Respite Care, and Routine Home Care.

Free-standing Hospice - see hospice house

GIP - General inpatient (GIP) care, one of the four levels of care mandated by the Medicare hospice benefit; if symptoms are too severe to be managed at home, a person hospice is cared for in a general inpatient (GIP) bed in a healthcare facility until symptoms are managed or under control. See Inpatient Care.

Graduate – Health improves for someone on hospice service to the point where they no longer qualify for hospice care. They are removed from service. See: revoke.

Grief - An emotional response to any loss.

Holistic Services - Special treatments (music therapy, massage, pet visits, reiki, acupuncture) that address the whole patient, not just the disease.

Home Hospice Care - See routine home care.

Home Medical Equipment - Supplies and equipment (hospital bed, wheelchair, patient lift equipment, oxygen and its delivery systems, bedside commode) that support the unique needs of an ill person at home.

Homelike Setting - a healthcare setting, as in a hospital or nursing home, that emphasizes art on the walls, colorful comforters on the beds and curtains at the windows, for example, rather than the clinical equipment, functionality and sterility of a typical hospital room.

Hospice - In America, a healthcare organization that gives care to the terminally ill. It focuses on comfort and quality of life rather than on curing the terminal disease. It often follows palliative care. In many countries around the world it is known as hospice.

Hospice Aide - A certified nursing assistant who provides personal or "custodial" care (help with eating, bathing, dressing, moving around, using the bathroom) near the end of life. *See nursing assisant.*

Hospice Care - comfort care (as opposed to curative care) that manages pain and symptoms so someone with a terminal illness can live each day to the fullest.

Hospice Care Team - Professional caregivers (RN, physician, social worker, chaplain, hospice aide, bereavement specialist and volunteer) who work together to care for the whole patient near the end of life. See Interdisciplinary Team.

Hospice Eligibility - Guidelines that determine if a person qualifies for the Medicare hospice benefit; two physicians, or one certified hospice doctor, must certify that the person has fewer than six months to live if the disease follows its usual course.

Hospice House - A building, usually freestanding, that is designated for the care of patients near the end of life and their families. See inpatient unit.

Hospice volunteers - Members of the community who donate their time and energy to perform tasks for a hospice, from visiting a terminally ill person to doing clerical work in the office. Medicare mandates that 5 percent of patient care must be performed by a local volunteer; hospice companies recruit volunteers and provide free training.

IDT - See interdisciplinary team.

Inpatient Care - One of the four levels of care mandated by the Medicare hospice benefit; around-the-clock care provided in a healthcare facility when the ill person's symptoms cannot be managed at home. The goal is to stabilize them so they can return to routine home care. See General Inpatient (GIP) Care.

Inpatient Unit - An area of a healthcare facility, often a floor or wing, dedicated exclusively to the care of patients near the end of life and their families. See hospice house.

Interdisciplinary Team (IDT) - The group of social workers, chaplains, nurses, Volunteer Manager, and several non-medical personnel who work together to care discuss the total care for each person on hospice service.

Living Will - A document that specifies what kind of medical treatment you would want if you had a terminal illness. It is called a "living" will because it directs what will happen to you while you are alive.

Medicare Hospice Benefit - Since 1982, Medicare has provided free medical and psycho-social services to anyone who has a doctor's order stating they have six months or less to live if their disease runs its expected course.

Mourning – A cultural response to loss.

Nurse Aide – Assist patients with their day to day care. There are also regional names for this area of medical care. *See nursing assistant.*

Nursing Assistant – assists patients with their day to day care. There are also regional names for this area of medical care. Also see nurse aide, CNA and STNA.

Palliative Care – In America, it is care given to the seriously ill person to address the symptoms of a chronic (incurable) illness. It is care that addresses every aspect of the person, not just the disease. It makes a disease or its symptoms less severe or unpleasant without removing the cause. It is comfort care. In many countries in the world, hospice care is called palliative care.

PCP – See Primary care physician.

Pickering House (PH) – FAIRHOPE's exclusive hospice house for general inpatient, respite and end of life care. See hospice house.

POC - plan of care; a document created by your hospice team that lists the services needed, the team member who will provide them, how often and what results are expected.

POA - See Power of Attorney

Power of attorney - (POA) power of attorney for healthcare. A document that identifies who will make healthcare decisions for you if you are unable to speak for yourself due to illness, injury or debilitation.

Primary care physician - (PCP) The personal physician who cares for you and refers you to specialists as necessary.

PRN – Abbreviation from the Latin phrase, "pro re nata". Depending on preference it means "as necessary" or "as the circumstance arises". Used frequently when dealing with the need for the use of pain medications.

Prognosis - The likely course of a disease or illness.

Recertification - A document that states who is receiving hospice services continues to be eligible beyond the allotted time of the last certification.

Referral – The suggestion that a certain person might be hospice eligible, usually made by a healthcare professional, but may also be made by non-professionals such as family or friends. It can begin with an evaluation and discussion that ends in admission to hospice.

Respite care - One of the four levels of care mandated by the Medicare hospice benefit. Used when the person receiving hospice care at home is temporarily transferred to a hospice house or an inpatient facility to provide up to five days of respite to the family caregiver.

Revoke – also commonly called revocation – a patient's choice to no longer receive hospice services through the Medicare Hospice Benefit. Patient must sign a statement expressing their wish to no longer exercise this benefit; he/she may readmit to hospice should their circumstances change at a later date.

Routine Home Care - One of the four levels of care mandated by the Medicare hospice benefit. It brings basic hospice services to wherever person lives.

Spiritual Care Coordinator – Provides direct spiritual support and counsel to the person on service and their family with respect to their belief system. Acts as a liaison between clergy of the local interfaith community and hospice.

STNA - State Tested Nursing Assistant. There are several regional terms for this area of medical care. See; CNA, Nurse Aide, Nursing Assistant.

Terminally Ill – Term used when a diagnosis of a disease or illness is that it cannot be cured; one that is expected to result in death in a short time.

Viewing – See: Calling Hours

Visitation – See: Calling Hours

Request for personal experiences

I am interested in learning about your experiences concerning hospice, whether as a volunteer, social worker, medical person or a member of the general staff. And I am also interested to hear from you if you have experienced hospice care through a family member or friend. And I am especially interested in hearing from you if you were on hospice service and your health improved--a surprisingly pleasant aspect of hospice care.

Please send your stories and experiences to:
Rick Schneider
P O Box 594
Lancaster, Ohio 43130

or

rickschneiderauthor@gmail.com

If your submission is included in the next book, you will be credited for your submission.

Rick

Index

Acceptance of illness, 23, 30, 61, 74
AIDS, 22, 144, 216
Alzheimer's Disease, 26
Ambulatory, 64, 152, 187
Anger, 66, 74, 99, 197, 215
Angels, 92, 159
Anniversaries, 154

Bedridden, 50, 86, 140, 144, 216
Before calling, 6, 9, 19, 68, 90
Bereavement, 171, 174

Calling Hours, 168
Calmness *(See also: Serenity)*, 31, 34, 60, 61, 64
Cancer, 187
Caregiver, Caregiving, 140, 143
Caregiver becomes unavaliable, 105, 108
Cats, *See: Pets*
Chaplain, 22, 36, 112, 159, 213
Child, Children, 168
C N A (Certified Nurse Assistant), *See: Nurse Assistant, Aide*
Comfort, Emotional, *See: Emotional Comfort*
Comfort, Physical, *See: Physical Comfort*
Comfort, Spiritual, See: Spiritual Comfort
Communication at end of life:
 -Verbal, 41, 66, 72, 176
 -Non Verbal, 86, 90, 96, 99, 144, 195
 -Consult, 19, 23, 36, 80
Control, Independence, *See: Independence, Control*
Courage, 96
Curative treatment, 6, 208

Daily routine, *(See also: Normalcy)*, 108, 116, 128, 144, 187
Daughter, 23, 96, 168
Dementia, 26
Disease:
 -appropriate for hospice, 22, 26, 45, 148, 213
 -Non-terminal related, 16, 208
Doctor, 77, 208
Dogs, *See: pets*
Dying Process, 224

Effects of hospice care on family, 31, 32, 60
Emotional comfort, 6, 12, 48, 168, 215
Emotional pain, 23, 28, 32, 36, 199, 215
Empathy, 110, 112, 184, 220

Family:
 -Doctor, 77, 208
 -Effects of illness on, 19, 22, 31, 54

237

-Involved with care, 12, 19, 90, 140
-relationships, 23, 96, 143, 176
Father, 22, 31, 86, 180, 205
Fear, 6, 9, 21, 40, 66
First call, 45, 56
Food, Importance at end of life, 99, 121, 124, 190, 206
For profit hospice, 28
Fundraising, 58, 182
Funeral, 168, 199

Giving possessions away, 61
Graduate from hospice care, *See: Sign off hospice*
Gratitude, 31, 34, 60, 202, 217
Grief:
   -Anticipatory, 90, 164, 168, 174, 199
   -Counselling, 13, 58, 168, 172, 174
   -Holidays, Special Days, 148, 171, 190, 199
   -Pets, 130

Haircut, Hair-do, 90, 144
Health improves, 40, 148, 152, 157, 187
Holidays, All, 182, 187, 189, 199
Hope, 16, 64, 96, 148, 217
Hospice appropriate, *See: disease, hospice appropriate*
Hospice doctor, 77
Hospice does:
   -Allow the ill person to sign off service, 148, 152, 157
   -Offer skilled nursing care, 13
   -Allow family control over care, 46, 90, 143

Hospice:
-does not cause death, 9, 40, 56, 82, 148
-service does not end at death, 103, 164, 168, 172, 174
-does not mean giving up hope, 40, 96, 148
-is not a continuation of curative care, 6,
-is not a place to go for care, 12, 58, 96, 103, 111
-is not expensive, 28, 54, 58, 174
-is not one National Organization, 9, 10, 28, 58
-is not just for the actively dying, 64, 96, 148, 187
-is not a continuance of medical care, 46, 60
-is not sad and depressing, 10, 12, 48, 96, 187
-is not only for old people, 22
-is not for 6 month or less exclusively, 9, 26, 64, 148
Hospice House, Facility, 128, 143, 190, 199, 215
Hospice overview, 10, 36, 58
Hospice types (Non-profit and for-profit), 9, 10, 54, 58
Hospital, Medical Facility, 41
How is hospice care provided?, 62
Humor, by those on service, 16, 74, 144
Humor, 75, 120, 140, 202

Independence, Control, 12, 48, 61, 111, 187
Individualized Care, 12, 46, 62, 66, 68, 144

238

Initial meeting with hospice staff, *See: Consult*

Kindness (*See also: Thoughtfulness*), 110, 144, 168, 190, 215

Last Hours:
 -Of life, 86, 90, 92, 135, 159, 220
 -Of life described, 224
Last Stage of Life, 50, 82, 159
Last Wishes, one more time wishes, 86, 99, 121, 148
Laundry, 108
Laughter, 120
Life expectancy, 40, 152, 157, 187
Life review, 80, 190, 199, 205
Location where care is given, *See: Where Hospice Care is Administered*

Married couple, 105, 107, 154, 195
Medical Facility, Hospital, 41
Medicare, 9, 54, 58
Medical equipment in the home, 12
Military, Veterans, 197, 199, 210
Mother, Mom, 23, 96, 126, 168

National hospice organization, 12, 28, 58
Non-medical staff, 164
Non-profit hospice, 28
Normalcy, 6, 12
Nurse, 22, 31, 68, 96, 103
Nurse Assistant, Aide, 99, 110, 120, 215

One more time wishes, last wishes, *See: Last Wishes*

Pain, Emotional, *See: Emotional Pain*
Pain, Physical, *See: Physical Pain*
Pain, Spiritual, *See: Spiritual Pain*
Palliative Care, 208
Parakeet, 132
Parent, 22, 96, 143, 168, 180
Peace (*See also: Serenity*), 34, 64
Pets:
 -Cats involved, 126, 128, 135
 -Dogs involved, 92, 132, 137, 139
Physical Comfort, 64, 216
Physical Pain, 23, 32, 205, 216
Pickering House, *See: Hospice House, Facility*
Plan of Care, 10, 80, 96, 187
Prayer, 16, 209
Purpose in Life, 40, 50, 64, 96, 172

Religion, 16, 36, 213
Revoke Care, *See: Sign off hospice*

Sad, 195
Serenity, (*See also: Peace*), 36, 40, 60, 96, 116
Sheltering Family from Upsetting news, 41
Sign off Hospice, 148, 152, 157
Sisters, 23, 90, 164
Social Worker, 22, 23, 80
Son, 22, 80, 86, 180
Specialist, 77
Spiritual Comfort, 36, 159, 164
Spiritual Event, 90, 219
Spiritual Leader, *See: Chaplain*

Spiritual Pain, 32, 36, 215
Spiritual Visions, *See: Visions, Spiritual*
Spirituality, Faith, 16, 90, 159, 164, 213, 216
Spouse, 105, 108, 171, 195, 199
STNA State Tested Nurse Assistant, *See: Nurse Assistant, Aide*

Thoughtfulness (*See also: Kindness*), 99, 103, 112, 194, 206, 215
Time to give to those on service, 103, 112, 210, 215
Types of hospice; Non-profit, for profit, 9, 10, 28, 58

Veterans, Military, 197, 199
Visions, Spiritual, 159
Visitation, *See: Calling Hours*
Volunteers, 66, 108, 116, 140, 144, 154, 203, 210

Wedding, Wedding Anniversary, 96
When is Hospice Appropriate, 26, 45, 50
Where is Hospice Care Administered, 12, 111
Who Administers Hospice Care, 62, 112, 116
Who May Refer Someone to Hospice, 183

www.ingramcontent.com/pod-product-compliance
Lightning Source LLC
LaVergne TN
LVHW011812060526
838200LV00053B/3743